Better Homes and Gardens®

GOOD FOOD & FITNESS

On the cover: *Lamb-Stuffed Squash,*
and *Orange Sponge Cake* (see index for
recipe pages).

**BETTER HOMES
AND GARDENS® BOOKS**
Editor: Gerald M. Knox
Art Director: Ernest Shelton
Food and Nutrition Editor: Doris Eby
Senior Food Editor: Sharyl Heiken
Senior Associate Food Editors: Sandra
    Granseth, Elizabeth Woolever
Associate Food Editors: Bonnie Lasater,
    Julia Martinusen, Marcia Stanley, Joy Taylor,
    Diana Tryon
Recipe Development Editor: Marion Viall
Test Kitchen Director: Sharon Golbert
Test Kitchen Home Economists: Jean Brekke,
    Kay Cargill, Marilyn Cornelius, Maryellyn
    Krantz, Marge Steenson
Associate Art Directors: Neoma Alt West,
    Randall Yontz
Copy and Production Editors: David Kirchner,
    Lamont Olson, David A. Walsh
Assistant Art Director: Harijs Priekulis
Senior Graphic Designer: Faith Berven
Graphic Designers: Alisann Dixon, Linda
    Ford, Tom Wegner

Editor in Chief: James A. Autry
Editorial Director: Neil Kuehnl
Group Administrative Editor: Duane Gregg
Executive Art Director: William J. Yates

Good Food & Fitness
Editor: Bonnie Lasater
Copy and Production Editor: Lamont Olson
Graphic Designer: Neoma Alt West
Consultant: Michael P. Scott

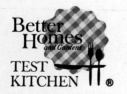

CONTENTS

GOOD FOOD
& FITNESS

Good food and fitness are two of the most often misunderstood but vital elements of a revolution that's been in progress for more than a decade.

Today, countless millions of Americans have chosen to actively pursue "wellness" life-styles that center around good nutrition and physical fitness. If you ask these health revolutionaries why, the answers are universally similar: Getting fit and staying fit makes them *look* better *feel* better, and best of all, *feel better about themselves.* For evidence, just ask anyone who regularly jogs, plays tennis, or skis cross-country.

The revolution is far from over, however. Instead of thinking in terms of good food and fitness, Americans tend to think in terms of "diet and exercise," which often brings to mind failed "miracle diet" schemes and endless, boring calisthenics. Most people have learned through experience that these are not productive.

It doesn't have to be so, and in the pages that follow are nutrition and exercise suggestions to make visible and positive changes in the way you look and feel.

But our good advice must be accompanied by a sincere commitment on your part to think of your diet and the level of activity in your life-style as a continuing lifelong process.

As countless "dieters" can tell you, nothing is more certain to fail in the long run than a crash diet. No sooner are the pounds off than they return.

There is really no drudgery involved in adopting sensible eating and exercise habits. You'll soon find out that it's just as easy to eat and exercise properly as it is not to. As your appearance and attitude improve, you'll soon find that exercise and a sensible pattern of eating are downright enjoyable.

All it takes is some careful thought about the kinds of food you eat, a liberal dose of will-power to stick to the first few weeks of exercises, and the knowledge that your life *will* become more enjoyable, and perhaps longer.

Furthermore, the example you set for others (especially your children) may help keep them healthier and happier for the rest of their lives, too.

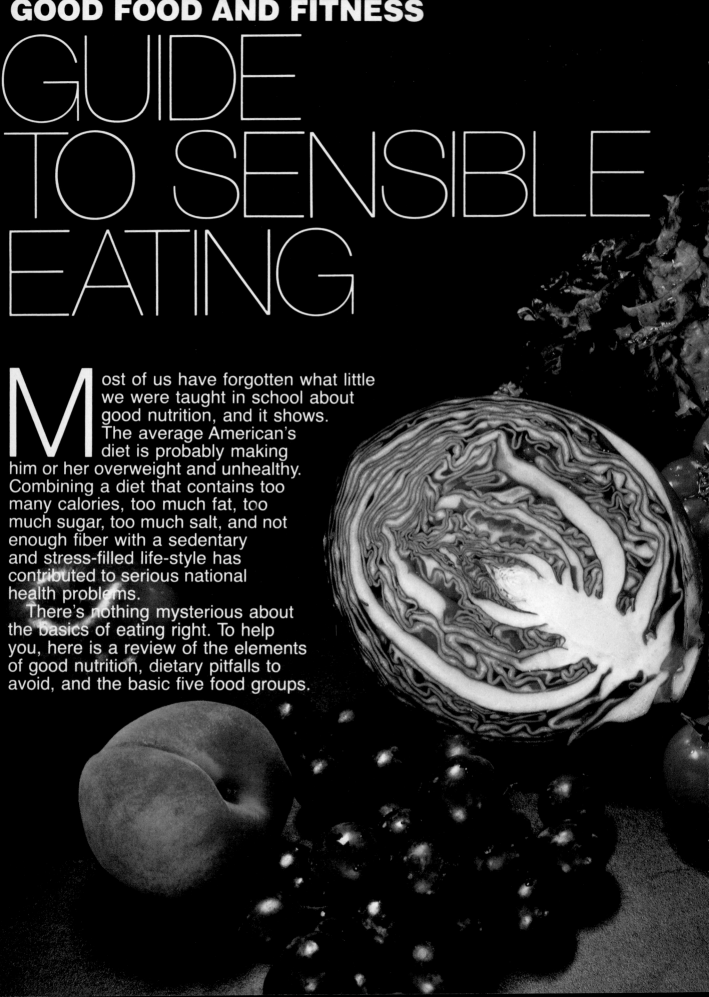

GUIDE TO SENSIBLE EATING

Most of us have forgotten what little we were taught in school about good nutrition, and it shows. The average American's diet is probably making him or her overweight and unhealthy. Combining a diet that contains too many calories, too much fat, too much sugar, too much salt, and not enough fiber with a sedentary and stress-filled life-style has contributed to serious national health problems.

There's nothing mysterious about the basics of eating right. To help you, here is a review of the elements of good nutrition, dietary pitfalls to avoid, and the basic five food groups.

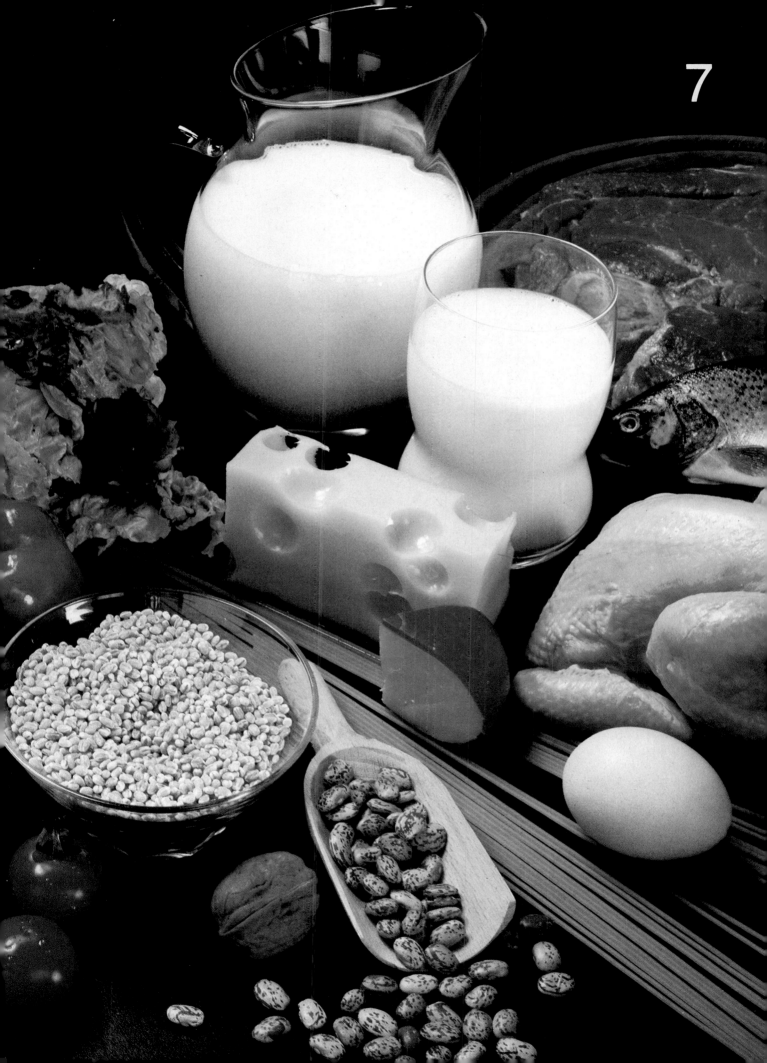

BASICS OF NUTRITION

Changing from a poor diet to one that's well balanced isn't difficult if you start by understanding the basics of good nutrition.

Basically, food is composed of proteins, carbohydrates, fats, vitamins, minerals, and water—about 50 essential nutrients in all. Most foods contain several of the basic nutrients, but no food has them all, so a balanced diet will include many kinds of foods. This variety ensures that eating right is anything but dull.

PROTEIN—THE BODY BUILDER

Protein is made up of building blocks called amino acids that are necessary to build, maintain, and repair the body. Protein is also involved in the production of healthy red blood cells, antibodies that prevent diseases, and hormones that regulate body functions.

With so much to do, protein supplies are quickly used up and need to be replenished frequently. Adults, teenagers, and children require about 65 grams of protein daily. Pregnant or nursing women need more.

Most of the body's energy comes from fats and carbohydrates, but when they aren't sufficient, protein can be used to supply energy. Too *much* protein in the diet is converted to body fat.

High quality protein sources supply all of the needed amino acids, including eight the body can't manufacture. These include meat, eggs, milk and cheeses, fish, and poultry.

Plant forms of protein such as dried beans and peas, whole grains and cereals, and nuts are of lesser quality, but they can be combined with high quality protein sources to make them nutritionally valuable. Macaroni and cheese is a good example because animal and plant proteins—milk, cheese, and enriched pasta—are combined.

FATS— CONCENTRATED ENERGY

It's hard to think of fats as being an essential or necessary part of a well-balanced diet, especially if you're trying to lose weight. Yet, fats in the diet make it possible for carbohydrates and proteins to be used to their best advantage.

Fats are highly concentrated forms of energy. They provide nine calories per gram compared to four calories per gram of protein and carbohydrate.

Fats transport vitamins A, D, E, and K into the body where they can be absorbed. A certain amount of fat makes food taste good, and because fats are digested slowly, they keep you from feeling hungry longer than do proteins or carbohydrates.

As you might expect, fat is a natural insulator and helps your body maintain its normal temperature.

The most common sources of fat in your diet probably are oils, butter, margarine, shortenings, and meat. But there are hidden sources of fats, too: baked products, fried foods, dressings, nuts, eggs, some milk products, and even lean meat.

Fats that are solid at room temperature are called *saturated* fats. *Unsaturated* fats are usually liquid. *Polyunsaturated* fats (such as safflower, corn, peanut, and soybean oils) are a chemical variation of unsaturated fats and contain essential elements that the body can't manufacture.

Some medical authorities believe that saturated fats tend to increase blood cholesterol levels. And some researchers say that high cholesterol plays an important role in heart disease. Others think its role has been overstated. That is why nutrition experts have issued conflicting advice about the types of fats and amount of cholesterol we should include in our diets.

Fat should make up one-fourth to one-third of the total calories you consume. Unless otherwise recommended by your doctor, eat moderate amounts of saturated and unsaturated fat.

CARBOHYDRATES— ENERGY FOR THE BODY'S WORK

Carbohydrates are another source of energy, but they're generally lower in calories than fats. They play an important role in the body's production of certain vitamins.

Carbohydrates are available in two basic forms: starches and sugars. They exist as *natural* sugars in fresh fruits, vegetables, and some dairy products. *Pure* or *refined* sugars such as honey, corn syrup, brown sugar, molasses, and table sugar also provide carbohydrates.

Foods such as potatoes, breads, cereals, and pasta are starch forms of carbohydrates.

Starches offer as much nutritional value as foods that contain natural sugars, but watch what you eat. Americans often combine fats with starchy foods (butter with potatoes, rich sauces with pasta). If you pay attention to the amount of fat in your diet, the starches aren't likely to cause undue problems. Another caution related to carbohydrates: Some diets call for severe restrictions in carbohydrate intake. When that happens, your body compensates by manufacturing energy from protein and creating a nutritional deficit. The trade-off—using valuable protein for energy— isn't worth it.

VITAMINS

Each of the 14 vitamins required by our bodies performs a specific function that no other nutrient can. Vitamins trigger the release of energy in your body, and regulate the way the body builds tissue and uses food.

Here's a capsule list of some of the more important vitamins:

• Vitamin A aids night vision and helps prevent eye disease, promotes bone growth in infants and children, and helps maintain the mucous membranes in the ears, nose, and intestinal lining. Leafy green and yellow vegetables, liver, apricots, cantaloupe, tomatoes, and dairy products are good sources.

• Thiamine (vitamin B_1) helps regulate your appetite, maintain a responsive nervous system, and release energy from carbohydrates. Thiamine is found in enriched cereals, whole grains, pork, nuts, and green peas.

• Riboflavin (another B vitamin) aids food metabolism, promotes healthy skin, and helps the body use oxygen. Milk, meats, eggs, dark green leafy vegetables, and whole grains are rich in riboflavin.

• Niacin (another B vitamin) is involved in fat metabolism, tissue respiration, and the conversion of sugars to energy. Liver, poultry, fish, nuts, enriched cereals, and peanut butter are good sources.

• Vitamin C (ascorbic acid) helps form collagen, the substance that binds body cells together. Vitamin C is essential to the growth and repair of teeth, gums, blood vessels, and specialized cells in the bones. You'll find vitamin C in citrus fruits, green leafy vegetables, strawberries, tomatoes, and potatoes.

MINERALS

Minerals play a crucial role in the body even though they occur in minute quantities.

Minerals aid blood coagulation, and without them vitamins would not be stimulated to action. Here are some of the more important minerals:

• Calcium, necessary for healthy bones and teeth, is present in dairy products, sardines, and enriched cereals.

• Phosphorus produces firm and supple skin, and is present in eggs, tuna, and bananas.

• Iron is essential for red blood cells to supply oxygen to the body. Meats, bran cereals, dried beans, prunes, and spinach provide iron.

The RDA (Recommended Daily Allowance), established for 15 of the 21 essential minerals, can be met if you eat a well-balanced diet.

WATER

Water isn't usually thought of as food, but it's essential to all tissues. In fact, our body weight is two-thirds water. You should drink seven glasses of water each day in addition to the water that's naturally in the foods you eat.

DIETARY RECOMMENDATIONS

Even when you know the basics of good nutrition, it's often hard to apply those principles unless you know just where you're going wrong and how to change your diet for the better.

A surgeon general of the United States has said Americans could be healthier if they would consume: only enough calories to meet their body's needs and to maintain an appropriate weight (or consume fewer calories if overweight); less saturated fat and cholesterol; less salt; less sugar; more complex carbohydrates such as whole grains, cereals, fruits, and vegetables; more fish, poultry, and legumes; and less red meat.

Add to those recommendations advice about consuming alcohol in moderate amounts, and you've got the basics of a nutritious lifelong eating plan.

EXCESSIVE CALORIES

Regardless of the foods we eat, most of us tend to eat too much. A calorie is simply a measure of the energy that can be derived from the body's processing of foods. One goal of a balanced diet is to match the number of calories you eat with the amount of energy you expend in your daily routine and through exercise.

If you're overweight, you're asking for trouble. Obesity is linked with high blood pressure, diabetes, heart attack, stroke, and increased fat and cholesterol levels in the blood.

TOO MUCH FAT IN THE DIET

Excessive fats (especially saturated fats) in the diet result in more than just being overweight: Some medical authorities say they're a prime contributor to high blood cholesterol in some people. Although fats provide energy and make foods taste better, some of us go overboard on them.

If you want to avoid excessive fats in your diet:

- Choose lean meat, fish, poultry, dried beans, and dried peas as sources of protein.
- Eat eggs and organ meats (such as liver) in moderate amounts.
- Limit the amount of butter, cream, shortenings, and foods made with those products.
- Trim excess fat from meats.
- Broil, bake, or steam your food instead of frying it whenever possible.

TOO MUCH SALT

Salt (or sodium), although tasty, contributes to the retention of body fluids and, as is the case with many other dietary excesses, is linked to high blood pressure and other diseases. Salt is present in almost any food you eat, but especially in processed foods. For example, there's enough salt in two slices of bread to meet your body's daily requirement for salt.

TOO MUCH SUGAR

It's estimated that the average American eats more than 130 pounds of sugar and other sweeteners each year. The havoc that plays with your teeth is obvious.

Although eating excessive amounts of sugar does not necessarily cause diabetes, and hasn't been linked to heart or blood vessel disease, sugar contributes little more than calories to your diet.

All too often, Americans substitute sugar calories for calories from other foods.

To cut back on sugar:

• Check labels on food products for other words that indicate the presence of sweeteners (sucrose, glucose, dextrose, fructose, corn syrups, or natural sweeteners).

• Eat fewer of the foods that contain lots of sugar: pies, cakes, cookies, sweet rolls, ice cream, soft drinks, candy.

• Substitute unsweetened fruit juices or water for soft drinks whenever possible.

• Use unsweetened cereals.

LACK OF FIBER

The evidence about the value of fiber in the diet is not yet conclusive, but many scientists believe the lack of fiber in the diet contributes to such problems as appendicitis, intestinal disorders, and gallstones.

Dietary fiber is a catchall term for a number of non-nutritive plant substances that can't be digested well by the body.

Most fiber comes from the structural parts of plants—the leaves, flowers, seeds, fruits, stems, and roots.

The most common fiber is cellulose, found in the cell walls of vegetables.

You can increase the amount of fiber in your diet by eating more foods made with whole grain (such as breads and cereals), bran, dried peas and dried beans, nuts, and fruits. Fruits and vegetables that have edible seeds, or which can be eaten unpeeled are among the best sources of fiber.

ALCOHOL IN MODERATION

Alcoholic beverages are high in calories, but contribute very little else to the diet.

Some evidence exists that an ounce or two of alcohol a day probably isn't harmful. But consumption of excessive amounts of alcohol often results in diminished appetite for other essential foods, and contributes to liver and neurological disorders and birth defects.

The best advice about drinking alcohol remains: Do so in moderation.

NUTRITIONAL LABELING

When you're grocery shopping and are confronted with literally thousands of food choices, how can you possibly know which foods contain the essential vitamins and minerals? Which foods are too high in salt, sugar, or fat? Ounce for ounce, which foods are highest in calories?

One handy source of dietary information is found on food labels themselves.

Since 1975, any food product with nutrients added and any for which nutritional claims are made must provide nutritional information on the label according to a standard format.

Even if not required by law to do so, many food companies label their food products voluntarily.

The Food and Drug Administration hopes that eventually all foods in the grocery store will be labeled so you can compare the nutritional value of the products just as you can now compare prices.

The information on nutrition labels is similar and includes the following:

• The number of calories and the gram weights of protein, fat, and carbohydrates must be listed for single serving amounts.

• The labels may show the amounts of cholesterol and salt (listed as sodium) in 100 grams of food, or per serving.

• The percentage of U.S. Recommended Daily Allowances (U.S. RDA) for protein and for seven vitamins and minerals (A, C, thiamine, riboflavin, niacin, calcium, and iron) must follow.

Any of 12 other nutrients must be listed when added by the food manufacturer.

• The label may include the amounts of polyunsaturated and saturated fats.

The U.S. RDAs reflect the highest amounts of various nutrients needed to meet the dietary needs of most *healthy* Americans.

BASIC FIVE FOOD GROUPS

Use these food groups to plan your daily calorie and nutrient requirements. Beware of foods in the fifth group. They contribute little more than calories to your diet.

Nutritionists have supplemented the basic four food groups you probably studied in school—fruits and vegetables; bread and cereals; milk and cheese; meat, poultry and fish—with a fifth one (fats, sweets, and alcohol). This important new category recognizes those foods that contain lots of calories, but have little other nutrient value. As you plan your diet, concentrate on using foods in the first four groups because of the nutrients and fiber they contain.

VEGETABLE-FRUIT GROUP

This group provides vitamins A and C, other nutrients, and fiber. Dark green and deep yellow vegetables are good sources of vitamin A. Vitamin C comes from dark green vegetables (if they're not overcooked), citrus fruits, melons, berries, and tomatoes, unpeeled fruits and vegetables, and foods with edible seeds.

Most vegetables and fruits are low in fat (two exceptions are olives and avocados), and none contain the cholesterol found in meats.

Recommended servings: 4 daily. Serving size: ½ cup counts as a serving. This might be one orange, half a medium grapefruit or cantaloupe, a wedge of lettuce, or a medium potato.

BREAD-CEREAL GROUP

These whole grain or enriched foods are important sources of iron, thiamine, niacin, and riboflavin.

Fortified breakfast cereals usually contain nutrients not normally found in cereals, such as vitamins B_{12}, C, and D.

Included in the bread-cereal group are all products made with whole grains, enriched flour or meal; bread, biscuits, muffins, waffles, cooked or ready-to-eat cereals, cornmeal, macaroni, spaghetti, noodles, rice, rolled oats, and barley.

Recommended servings: 4 daily. Serving size: 1 slice of bread; ½ to ¾ cup cooked cereal, macaroni, noodles, or rice, or 1 ounce ready-to-eat cereal.

MILK-CHEESE GROUP

These foods (including low-fat or skim milk products) are major sources of calcium. They also add riboflavin, protein, and vitamins A, B_6, B_{12}, and usually are fortified with vitamin D. Milk and cheese aren't the only beneficial foods in this group. Also choose yogurt, ice milk, cottage cheese, buttermilk, and any other form of milk.

Recommended daily servings: Children 9 to 12: 3 servings; teens: 4 servings; adults: 2 servings; pregnant women: 3 servings; nursing mothers: 4 servings.

Serving size: One cup (8 ounces) of milk counts as a serving. Also: 1 cup plain yogurt; 1⅓ ounces hard cheese; 1½ cups ice milk; ¼ cup Parmesan cheese; 2 cups cottage cheese.

MEAT, POULTRY, FISH, BEANS, AND NUTS GROUP

This group supplies protein, iron, thiamine, niacin, and riboflavin. Foods in this group such as meat and egg yolks also contain cholesterol. Fish and shellfish (with some exceptions) are relatively low in cholesterol.

Other foods in the group include dried beans or peas, soybeans, lentils, seeds, nuts, peanuts, and peanut butter.

Recommended daily servings: 2, vary sources.

Serving size: 2 to 3 ounces of lean, cooked meat, poultry, or fish, all without bone; two eggs, 1 cup cooked dried beans, peas, soybeans, or lentils. Or use ¼ cup peanut butter, ¼ to ½ cup nuts, sesame seeds, or sunflower seeds to count as one ounce of meat, poultry, or fish.

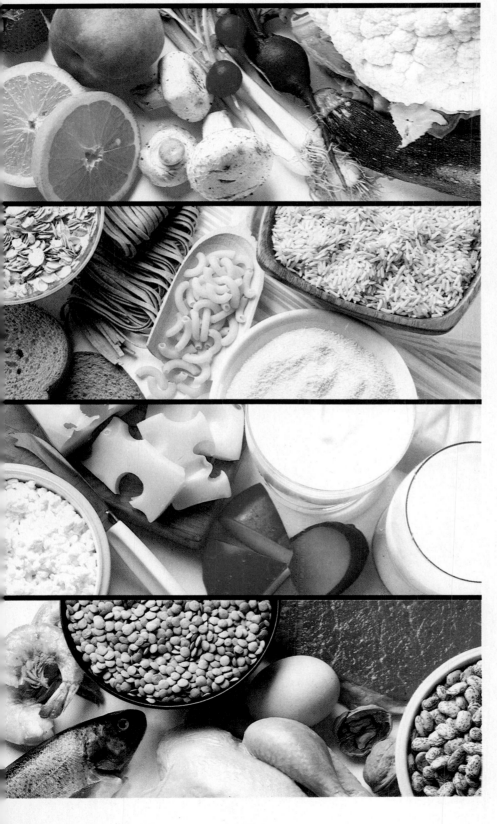

FATS, SWEETS, ALCOHOL GROUP

Be judicious about selecting foods from this group, because they are extremely high in calories. Unenriched, refined bakery goods are included because they provide relatively low levels of vitamins, minerals, and protein per calorie consumed. Other foods in the group are butter, margarine, mayonnaise, salad dressings, candy, sugar, jams, jellies, syrups, soft drinks, wine, beer, and other alcoholic beverages. To repeat: Go easy on these foods.

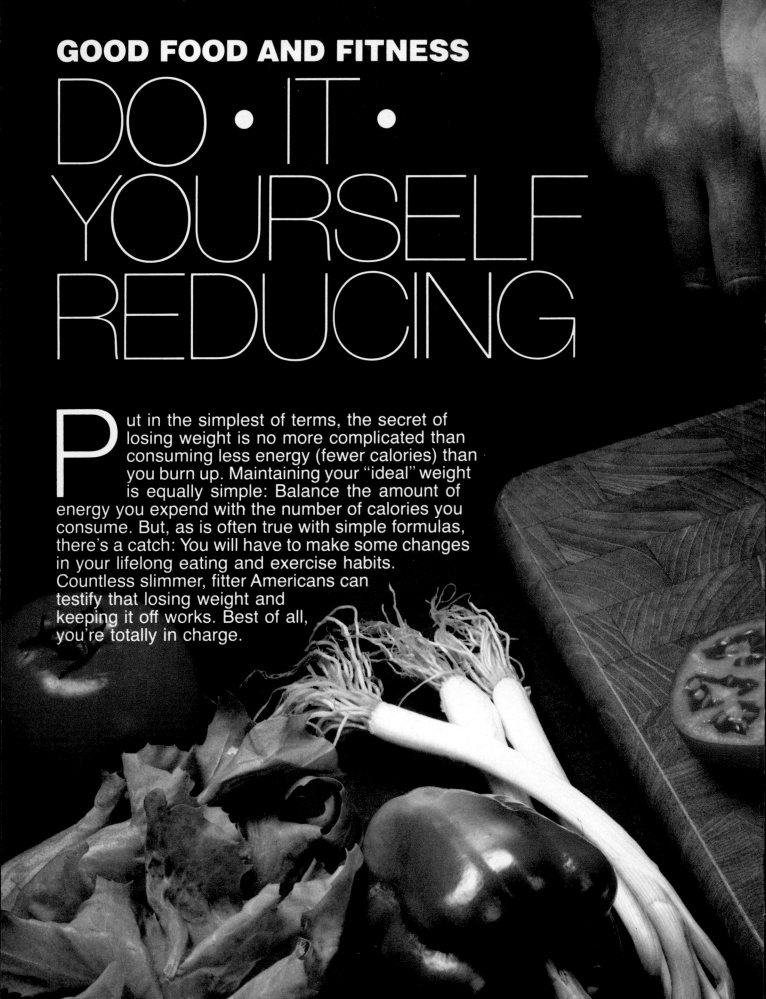

DO · IT · YOURSELF REDUCING

P ut in the simplest of terms, the secret of losing weight is no more complicated than consuming less energy (fewer calories) than you burn up. Maintaining your "ideal" weight is equally simple: Balance the amount of energy you expend with the number of calories you consume. But, as is often true with simple formulas, there's a catch: You will have to make some changes in your lifelong eating and exercise habits. Countless slimmer, fitter Americans can testify that losing weight and keeping it off works. Best of all, you're totally in charge.

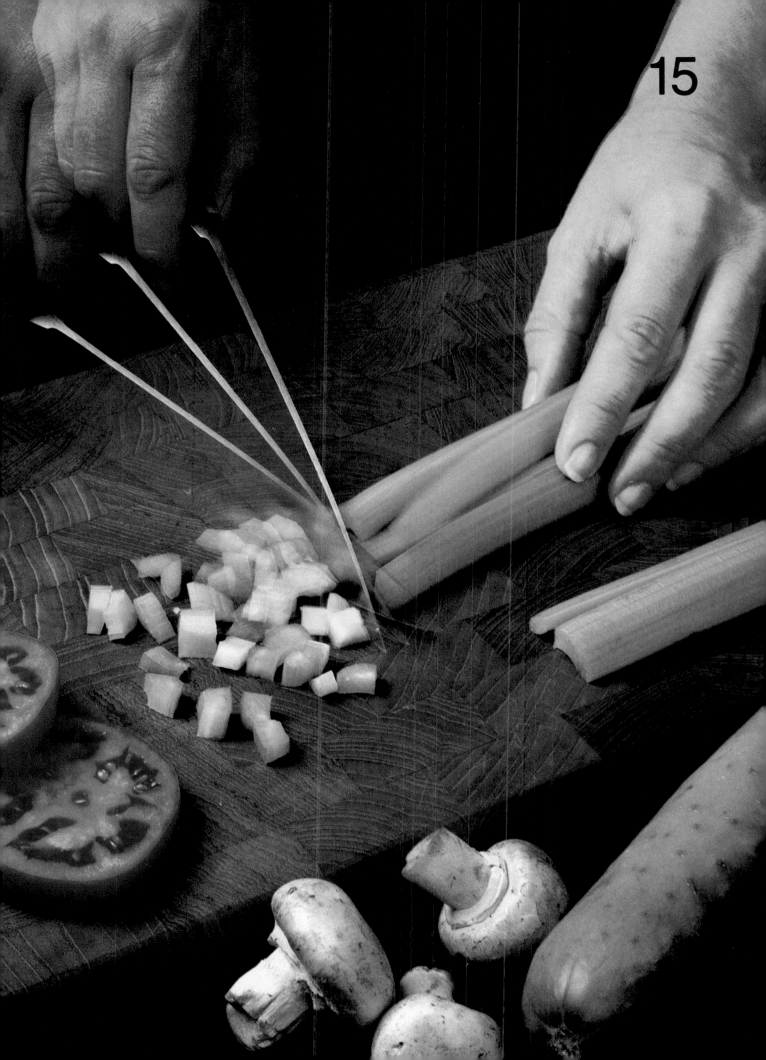

BEHAVIOR MODIFICATION

Successful dieters quickly realize they were eating more from habit, to relieve stress, or because of social custom than to meet the body's energy needs.

Whatever the cause of your weight problem, you should be able to apply some, if not all, of these proven dieting tips as you start to change why and when you eat:

• *Keep a meal record.* Before you begin to change the way you eat, keep a record for a week or two of what, when, where, and how much you eat. (A small notebook is handy for such record keeping.) Then, use a calorie chart (available in most bookstores) to figure out your daily caloric intake.

Total energy needs vary from person to person, but the chart on page 19 will help you approximate your ideal weight.

• *Identify the trouble spots and work on them.* After studying your diet record, look for ways to make changes. Have you acquired the habit of skipping meals, then gorging later to compensate? Are you snacking on high-calorie foods? Do you eat only to be sociable? Do you eat automatically, even if you're not really hungry?

Can you spot extra calories that can be eliminated without much hassle? If so, you're ready to change the why, when, and where of your eating habits by modifying your behavior.

Many of us are overweight because we associate eating with certain "cues" such as specific times of the day (coffee breaks, for instance), a particular mood (depression or boredom), even certain television commercials.

Behavior modification—the commonsense approach to dieting—teaches you to recognize your own cues and replace them with other forms of behavior. For instance, instead of eating while watching television, try knitting. Try substituting a good, brisk walk for a snack if you're bored or depressed.

• *Eat less, but more frequently.* If your record shows you're eating three big meals a day, you may want to change your eating pattern. Instead of a big breakfast, lunch, and dinner, reduce the size of each meal. Between meals, substitute low-calorie snacks. By doing so, you cut back on the total number of calories you consume, and still avoid feeling hungry all the time.

• *Use smaller plates.* Like many people, you're probably conditioned to clean every bit of food from your plate. And like many of us, you're probably overfilling your plate. So by limiting the size of the plate, you also limit the amount of food you consume at one sitting. By using smaller plates, you are still able to eat everything on it, only now the plate contains less food.

• *Change your snacking habits.* Substitute low-calorie foods for cookies, cakes, candy, and other traditional, high-calorie snacks. Fresh fruit and vegetables will satisfy your craving to munch, yet contribute few calories to your daily total.

• **Eat slowly.** Doing so allows your brain time to register the food you eat and stop the impulses that make you think you're hungry. By eating fast you override the brain-to-stomach circuitry that tells you when to quit. You become full—and overfull—before the brain can turn off the desire to eat. By eating slowly, you know when to quit and can easily employ one of the best dieting exercises: pushing yourself away from the table.

• **Use positive reminders.** One expert says (and only partly in jest) that the reason most diets fail is a subliminal, negative association with the first three letters in the word diet. Instead, try using the mnemonic "Think." The first four letters spell "thin;" the middle letter is "I." This, "I think thin" becomes an easy-to-remember, positive memory device to help you change your eating habits. And here's a gimmick to avoid because of the negative associations. Don't paste a picture of a fat person on the refrigerator door. Instead, find a photo of a person who looks like you'd *like* to look and post it in a variety of locations. Today, the photo might be on the refrigerator door, two days later move it to the mirror in your bathroom, then to the clothes closet, your car, and to the top of the TV set. This constant shuffling simply keeps a positive image of your eventual goal in front of you all the time.

HOW TO MAKE IT WORK

Here's a step-by-step guide to assuring success with your weight reduction program:

• **Ask for help if you need it.** You can begin a weight reducing diet by yourself, but if you're low on willpower, ask for help from your family doctor, friends, or one of the many reputable dieting organizations such as Weight Watchers, The Diet Workshop, TOPS (Take Off Pounds Sensibly), or Overeaters Anonymous.

• **Resolve to take it slow and easy.** The surest way to fail at losing weight is to set unrealistic goals. No doubt it took a considerable amount of time to put on those pounds, and it'll take time (but not as much) to get them off. Medical authorities recommend a weight loss goal of no more than two pounds a week.

• **Keep a written record of your progress.** This will help you evaluate your success at periodic intervals.

• **Prepare for some setbacks.** Losing weight is sometimes hard work. Don't worry if you suddenly find you've put a few pounds back on. Take heart that you've progressed as far as you have. Even if there are temporary setbacks, it probably won't seem as difficult to relose those few extra pounds as it did when you began.

• **Schedule rewards for yourself along the way.** For instance, the first time you're able to wear a smaller size, buy a new outfit. Your friends will notice the change and their compliments will be further impetus to continue your diet.

FAD DIETS— DO THEY WORK?

Fad diets, including fasting, or modified fasting, one-emphasis diets such as the so called "grapefruit" diet, and low carbohydrate, low protein, or high fiber diets, can be dangerous because they often restrict or eliminate many essential nutrients necessary for a nutritionally balanced diet. Often such fad diets are "rapid weight loss" schemes that seldom prove successful for more than a short time.

In fact, the up and down, roller coaster effect of repeated weight loss and gain may have more serious repercussions than maintaining a consistent weight, even if it is excessive.

The best dieting advice is to stay away from quick weight loss schemes, and stick to a diet that:

• Provides all the necessary nutrients but supplies fewer calories than you're now consuming.

• Includes foods from each of the basic five food groups, with only limited choices from the fats-sweets-alcohol group.

• Conforms to your individual tastes, habits, and budget.

• Doesn't leave you continually hungry, tired, and irritable.

• Is easy to follow both at home and away from home without making you feel "different" from others.

• Helps you learn eating habits you can continue for the rest of your life.

CALORIC NEEDS

To estimate the number of calories needed to keep your weight at its ideal level (see the height and weight chart on the opposite page), multiply your desired weight by 15 (multiply by 12 if you lead a less-than-active life). That gives you the approximate number of daily calories needed to maintain that weight.

If you're over (or under) your ideal weight, you're going to have to reduce or increase your caloric intake accordingly.

It takes 3,500 calories to make one pound of fat, so if you want to lose two pounds a week, you'll have to take in about 1,000 fewer calories per day than you burn up. Or you can decrease your caloric intake by 500 calories per day and exercise enough to burn the remaining 500.

t's no secret that excess pounds and inches have a tendency to mysteriously creep up on us all. No doubt you've heard it said (or said it yourself): "I don't eat any more than I ever did, and I *still* put on weight."

The mystery evaporates when you study lifetime exercise and work habits. In that first job out of school, you may have been in a position that required manual labor or considerable activity.

Then, as your experience and knowledge increased, your job changed from "doing" to managing. You probably *aren't* eating more than you did, but your activity level has been reduced and you're burning up fewer calories.

The tip at the top of this column tells how to estimate the number of calories you need daily to maintain your ideal weight.

The President's Council on Physical Fitness says that lack of physical activity is more often the cause of overweight than is overeating. The council cites lack of exercise as the most important cause of the "creeping" obesity in our mechanized society.

Put another way, with no increase in activity just one extra can of cola, an extra slice of buttered bread, or anything else that adds about 100 calories to your diet each day can add up to 10 extra pounds a year.

But, if you skip those extra calories and walk an extra mile each day, you'll take off those excess pounds in a year.

Moreover, exercise has benefits beyond weight loss. You'll look better, tone up flabby muscles, sleep better, and be better equipped to take life's frustrations in stride.

The chart on this page gives you a good idea of the number of calories expended (per hour) by a 150-pound person in various activities. The heavier you are, the more energy you expend for each activity because you also have to expend more energy just to move yourself around.

It's apparent that there's energy expenditure in everything you do, even sleeping. But your excess pounds will come off more quickly if you look for ways to increase the amount of energy you burn in activities that are pleasant to you, such as gardening, bicycling, walking, or even mowing the lawn.

Energy expended (per hour) by a 150-pound person in various activities

Activities	Calories Burned Per Hour
Rest and Light Activity	50-200
Lying down or sleeping	80
Sitting	100
Driving an automobile	120
Standing	140
Domestic work	180
Moderate Activity	200-350
Bicycling (5½ mph)	210
Walking (2½ mph)	210
Gardening	220
Canoeing (2½ mph)	230
Golf	250
Lawn Mowing (power mower)	250
Bowling	270
Lawn Mowing (hand mower)	270
Fencing	300
Rowboating (2½ mph)	300
Swimming (¼ mph)	300
Walking (3¾ mph)	300
Badminton	350
Horseback riding (trotting)	350
Square dancing	350
Volleyball	350
Roller skating	350
Vigorous Activity	over 350
Table tennis	360
Ditch digging (hand shovel)	400
Ice skating (10 mph)	400
Wood chopping or sawing	400
Tennis	420
Water skiing	480
Hill climbing (100 ft. per hr.)	490
Skiing (10 mph)	600
Squash and handball	600
Cycling (13 mph)	660
Scull rowing (race)	840
Running (10 mph)	900

HEIGHT AND WEIGHT CHART

MEN *Acceptable Weight Range* (pounds)*

HEIGHT*	SMALL FRAME	MEDIUM FRAME	LARGE FRAME
5' 2"	112	123	141
5' 3"	115	127	144
5' 4"	118	130	148
5' 5"	121	133	152
5' 6"	124	136	156
5' 7"	128	140	161
5' 8"	132	145	166
5' 9"	136	149	170
5'10"	140	153	174
5'11"	144	158	179
6' 0"	148	162	184
6' 1"	152	166	189
6' 2"	156	171	194

WOMEN *Acceptable Weight Range* (pounds)*

HEIGHT*	SMALL FRAME	MEDIUM FRAME	LARGE FRAME
4'10"	92	102	119
4'11"	94	104	122
5' 0"	96	107	125
5' 1"	99	110	128
5' 2"	102	113	131
5' 3"	105	116	134
5' 4"	108	120	138
5' 5"	111	123	142
5' 6"	114	128	146
5' 7"	118	132	150
5' 8"	122	136	154
5' 9"	126	140	158
5'10"	130	144	163

This handy height and weight chart can tell you at a glance whether you need to gain or lose weight. The figures are averages, so your own ideal weight may vary by a few pounds.

*Height without shoes, weight without clothes

DO-IT-YOURSELF MENU PLANNING

A personalized, well-balanced and calorie-controlled eating plan is important in any reducing diet that produces lasting results. True, it doesn't offer the quick-and-easy solutions promised by many fad diets. There's no gimmick involved, no magic formula to follow, and no secret combination of foods. What it does provide is a commonsense approach to the problem of keeping your weight under control.

Getting to know your eating habits is the first step in putting together a custom-made eating plan aimed at reducing your weight. Your food likes, dislikes, and your particular way of life affect what, when, where, and how much you eat. Take a close look at your eating habits by keeping a record for one to two weeks of the types and amounts of foods you eat. Figure your daily calorie intake using a calorie chart (available at book stores).

After going through your completed inventory, check to see if the number of calories you've been consuming is the amount you require for your daily activities. (See page 18 for determining your calorie requirements.) If you take in more calories than you need, the excess will be stored as fat. To lose, you'll need to lower your calorie intake or exercise more.

Devising a calorie-reduced eating plan that is well-balanced may sound complicated, but it doesn't require you to be a nutrition expert. If it's well-balanced you'll find the weight easier to keep off, because the variety provided will help you stay with it.

To achieve a balanced diet, you must combine the right amounts from each of the basic food groups. The chart on pages 12 and 13 outlines the types of foods that belong in each group, the nutrients they supply, and the suggested number of daily servings. This basic food group system takes into account the RDA (Recommended Dietary Allowance), which is a nutritional standard set by the Food and Nutrition Board of the U.S. government. The RDA tells how much of the known nutrients are recommended to meet the needs of a healthy person. Each food group contains foods of similar nutrient content. By planning your meals to include the suggested number of servings from each essential group, you'll receive an adequate intake of nutrients. If you have any medical problems that may require a special diet, be sure to consult your doctor.

A MENU PLAN FOR YOU

Plan your meal schedule taking into account the demands of your day. If a traditional three-meal plan doesn't fit in, try a meal pattern that works better for you. Decide the number of meals you want per day, and the types of food you want to eat at certain times of the day. Consider each day's menu as a whole, keeping in mind the total calorie and nutrient content of the food. Begin your planning around a protein main dish from the meat group. Everyone requires 2 servings a day from the meat group. Pregnant women and nursing mothers need more. On a traditional three-meal plan you could serve a food from this group at two of the meals. If you're using a five-meal plan you could distribute the protein throughout the day by serving half portions at four of the meals. Next choose four servings from the fruit and vegetable group and four from the bread and cereal group. Servings from the milk group vary. Children need three servings, teenagers require four servings, and adults two servings. Work the required number of servings into the number of daily meals that you have chosen.

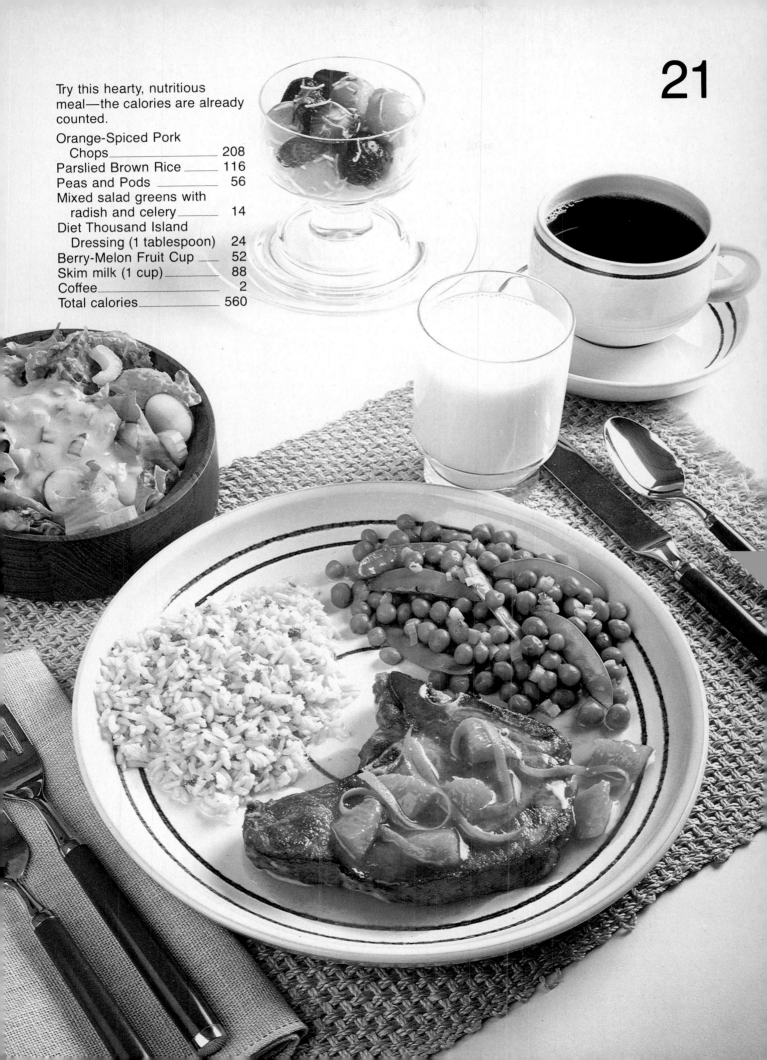

Try this hearty, nutritious meal—the calories are already counted.

SELECT-A-FOOD MENU PLANNER

Two generic menu plans are given at the right. One plan uses the usual three-meal-a-day schedule with snacks. The other is a five-meal plan. Simply plug in foods of your choice, keeping in mind your total calorie intake. By choosing low calorie foods from each of the four required food groups you can establish a well-balanced eating plan that helps you lose weight. Remember, the plan is flexible. Any servings from these four required food groups can serve as snacks or mini-meals, too.

OPTIONAL EXTRAS

Notice that the fats, sweets, and alcohol group is not included in the menu planner. This group contains foods that aren't required in your diet, so no recommended number of servings is given. Foods in this group mainly supply calories in far greater proportions than their nutrient value. These foods should be used in your diet only as your caloric allowances permit, providing that they don't replace foods from the four required groups.

AN EYE FOR SERVING SIZE

It's important to follow the serving sizes given in the Basic Five Food Groups Chart (pages 12 and 13). Train yourself to recognize the recommended serving size by weighing or measuring foods to see what an actual serving size looks like. The suggested amounts may seem small at first, but, in a short time you'll be able to estimate the correct serving size without going overboard.

3-MEAL PLAN

Meal 1
1 milk serving
1 citrus fruit serving
1 bread/cereal serving

Meal 2
1 meat serving
1 vegetable serving
1 bread/cereal serving

Snack
1 milk serving (*children and teenagers*)
1 bread/cereal serving

Meal 3
1 meat serving
1 vegetable serving (*deep green or yellow variety every other day*)
1 bread/cereal serving
1 fruit serving
1 milk serving

Snack
1 milk serving (*for teenagers*)

5-MEAL PLAN

Meal 1
1 milk serving
1 bread/cereal serving

Meal 2
½ meat serving
1 citrus fruit serving
1 bread/cereal serving

Meal 3
½ meat serving
1 milk serving
1 vegetable serving (*deep green or yellow variety every other day*)

Meal 4
1 milk serving (*for children and teenagers*)
1 vegetable serving
1 bread/cereal serving

Meal 5
1 meat serving
1 milk serving (*for teenagers*)
1 bread/cereal serving
1 fruit serving

SELECT-A-FOOD SAMPLE MENUS

The two sample menus below are based on the *Select-A-Food Menu Planner* (opposite). Use them to help you start planning a balanced, low-calorie eating plan. Recipes for items marked with an asterisk (*) are given in chapter 4 (see index for page numbers).

	BASIC FOOD GROUPS (number of servings)	SAMPLE 3-MEAL PLAN
MEAL 1	Milk (1)	1 cup skim milk
	Fruit/Vegetable (1)	½ grapefruit
	Bread/Cereal (1)	½ cup cooked oatmeal
MEAL 2	Meat (1), Bread/Cereal (1), and Fruit/Vegetable (½)	Beef and Sprout Sandwiches*
	Fruit/Vegetable (½)	3 carrot sticks (3 inch)
SNACK	Milk (1)	1 ounce mozzarella cheese (*children and teenagers*)
	Bread/Cereal (1)	1 English muffin, toasted
MEAL 3	Meat (1) and Fruit/Vegetable (1)	Sole Florentine*
	Bread/Cereal (1)	1 slice whole wheat bread
	Fruit/Vegetable (1)	Fruit Medley Salad*
	Milk (¼)	Orange Yogurt Pie*
	Milk (¾)	¾ cup skim milk
	Fats/Sweets/Alcohol	1 teaspoon butter
SNACK	Milk (1)	1 cup cocoa—made with skim milk (*teenagers*)
TOTALS	Meat	2 servings
	Fruit/Vegetable	4 servings
	Bread/Cereal	4 servings
	Milk	2 servings (3 for children, 4 for teenagers)
	Calories	1344

	BASIC FOOD GROUPS (number of servings)	SAMPLE 5-MEAL PLAN
MEAL 1	Milk (1)	1 cup fruit-flavored yogurt
	Bread/Cereal (1)	1 English muffin, toasted
	Fats/Sweets/Alcohol	1 teaspoon butter
	Fats/Sweets/Alcohol	2 teaspoons jelly
MEAL 2	Meat (½), Bread/Cereal (1), and Fats/Sweets/Alcohol	Open-face sandwich: 1½ ounces cooked chicken breast (sliced), 1 slice whole wheat toast, and 1 tablespoon low-calorie mayonnaise
	Fruit/Vegetable (1)	1 orange
MEAL 3	Fruit/Vegetable (1), Meat (½), and Milk (½)	Cottage Tomato Cups*
	Milk (½)	½ ounce cheddar cheese
MEAL 4	Fruit/Vegetable (1)	Garden Vegetable Dip* (½ cup vegetable dippers and ¼ cup dip)
	Bread/Cereal (1)	3 rye wafers
	Milk (1)	1 cup skim milk (*children and teenagers*)
MEAL 5	Meat (1) and Bread/Cereal (1)	Veal Sauté with Mushrooms*
	Fruit/Vegetable (1)	Fruit with Creamy Banana Dressing*
	Milk (½)	Mandarin Rice Pudding* (*teenagers,*)
	Milk (½)	½ cup skim milk (*teenagers*)
TOTALS	Meat	2 servings
	Fruit/Vegetable	4 servings
	Bread/Cereal	4 servings
	Milk	2 servings (3 for children, 4 for teenagers)
	Calories	1606

GUIDE TO GOOD FITNESS

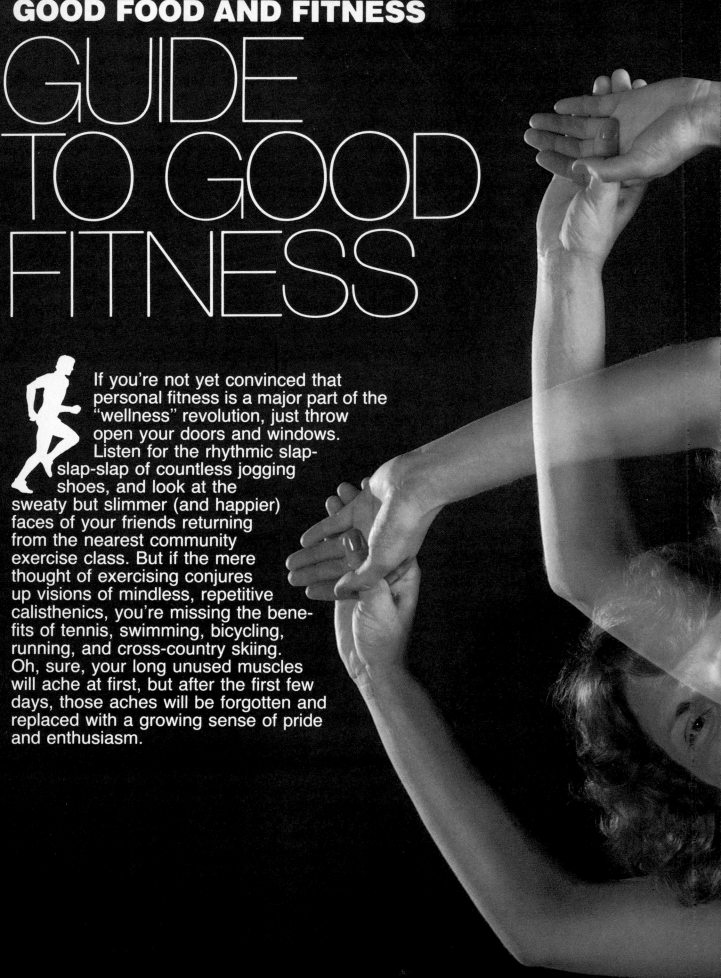

If you're not yet convinced that personal fitness is a major part of the "wellness" revolution, just throw open your doors and windows. Listen for the rhythmic slap-slap-slap of countless jogging shoes, and look at the sweaty but slimmer (and happier) faces of your friends returning from the nearest community exercise class. But if the mere thought of exercising conjures up visions of mindless, repetitive calisthenics, you're missing the benefits of tennis, swimming, bicycling, running, and cross-country skiing. Oh, sure, your long unused muscles will ache at first, but after the first few days, those aches will be forgotten and replaced with a growing sense of pride and enthusiasm.

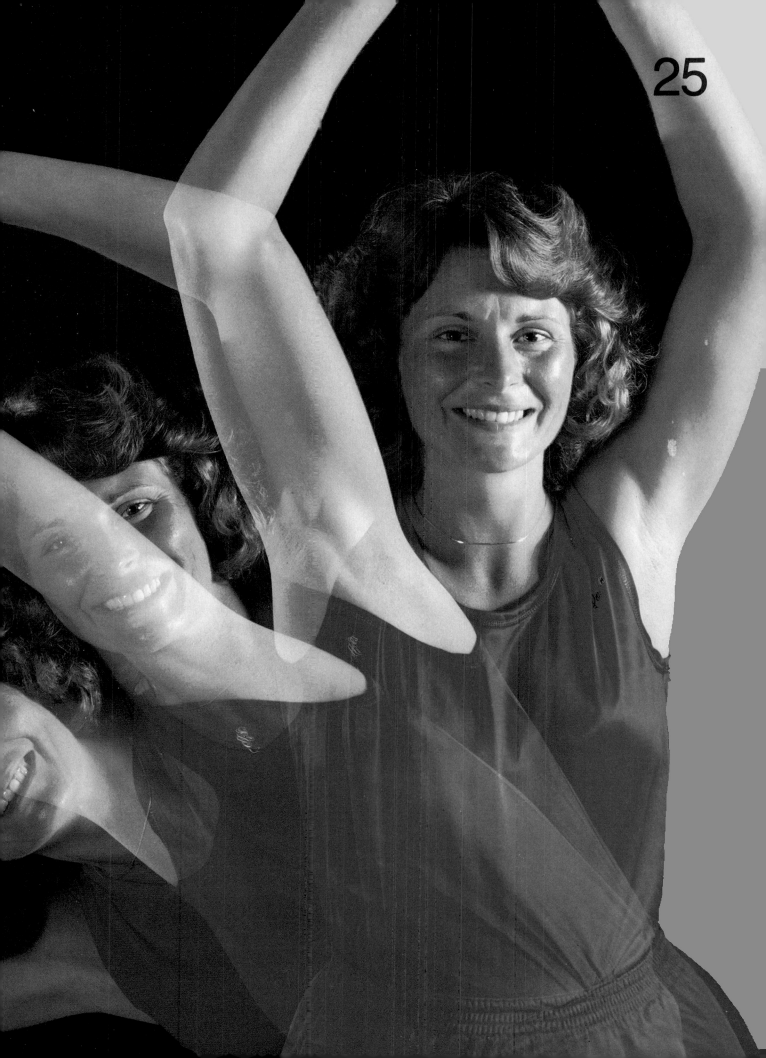

PLAN YOUR PROGRAM

Before you start to exercise, plan what you want to accomplish and how to go about it. Your decisions will depend on your present physical condition and your life-style.

No exercise program will transform an overweight, out of shape, lethargic person overnight. It took years for you to get out of shape, and it will take time to get back in shape. Here are some questions that need answers before you begin:
• Is your exercise program compatible with your physical condition? If you're a great deal overweight, or have a health problem such as hypertension, diabetes, or heart disease, check with your doctor before you start.
• Does a particular exercise suit the purpose that you have in mind? Do you want to get back in shape and stay there? Do you want to lose some weight and firm up some flabby muscles? Is one of your goals to combine exercise with fun? The options on page 27 will help you make the decision.

• Will your program of exercise enhance your overall physical condition? No matter what your ultimate goal, be sure to include exercises to strengthen your heart and improve your respiratory efficiency.
• Will it fit your schedule? Plan realistically. If you overestimate the time you have for exercise, you'll soon be backsliding. You may have to make some adjustments in your schedule, but even a comprehensive exercise program requires less than an hour each day to be effective, and 15 to 30 minutes of exercise three times a week is far more beneficial than no exercise at all.
• Will you enjoy it? If the thought of solitary early morning jogging turns you off, check out group exercise programs. Conversely, if competitive sports aren't appealing, you're a candidate for an exercise program with built-in solitary activities.

MISCONCEPTIONS ABOUT EXERCISE

Even if you have a physical condition that you *think* will keep you from exercising, chances are there's an exercise routine that would be good for you.

Here are the most common misconceptions about exercise.
• *It increases the appetite.* The truth is, surprisingly, that exercise before mealtime can decrease your appetite.
• *Exercise must be exhausting to be beneficial.* Not at all. You should work up a good sweat and be breathing hard if exercise is to do you any good. A good program gives your heart and lungs a sustained workout for 15 minutes but doesn't tax them to capacity.
• *Exercise is risky for persons over age 40 and isn't needed at all for the elderly.* Exercise is seldom risky for a healthy person who is accustomed to it, regardless of age. But if you're approaching middle age or haven't exercised before, get a medical checkup before you begin, and resist the temptation to keep up with the "youngsters."

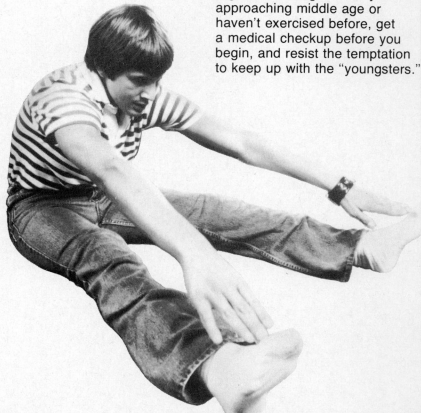

EXERCISE OPTIONS

Take your pick from an exercise menu that's as varied as can be. You'll find there's a type of exercise that is "custom made" just for you.

America's perception of the physically fit person has changed over the past few years. The burly football player's position as the epitome of fitness has been superceded by a downright skinny marathon runner, or a lean gymnast.

Of course, you don't have to be a marathon runner to be "in shape." Today there are lots of exercises designed to achieve physical fitness including aerobic dancing, cross-country skiing, volleyball, and soccer.

But no matter how you get there, the ultimate goal of fitness is to have healthy, efficiently functioning heart and lungs, muscular strength, flexible joints, agility, coordination, and a reserve of endurance and stamina.

FOUR MAJOR TYPES OF EXERCISE

Exercises are generally classified in one (or a combination) of the following four categories: isometric, isotonic, anaerobic, and aerobic.

• *Isometric exercises* increase the size and strength of muscles by tensing one set of muscles against another, or against an immovable object. Pushing against opposite sides of a doorjamb is an example.

• *Isotonic exercises* increase muscular strength, agility, coordination, and joint flexibility by repetitive contraction and relaxation of muscles. Weight lifting and calisthenics are examples.

• *Anaerobic exercises* build up stamina by demanding maximum energy output for brief periods of time. Examples are a 100-yard dash or a bicycle sprint.

• *Aerobic exercises* tone up the body and build heart and lung endurance by subjecting the body to sustained vigorous activity, such as swimming, running, or aerobic dancing.

If you want to be serious about exercise, and to get the most benefit from whichever program you choose, include at least one aerobic exercise in your daily routine.

TEAM AND INDIVIDUAL SPORTS

You can choose from a variety of sports exercise options, from group activities such as team sports to solitary activities such as running or swimming. You can also choose activities such as aerobic dancing that are not strictly defined as sports, but still fulfill the heart and lung exercise requirements needed to become physically fit.

Vigorous individual sports such as tennis, racquetball, and handball can be played for fun, as meaningful exercise, or both. The style of play you choose determines whether these, or any sport, will be of benefit. Each combines physical activity with companionship, is inexpensive, requires little in the way of athletic equipment, and can be just plain fun.

Individual sports are excellent for developing agility, reaction time, speed, and coordination.

Vigorous team sports, such as basketball, volleyball, baseball, touch football, softball, soccer, and field hockey are characterized by alternating periods of intense and relaxed play. Such sports can be considered a form of aerobic exercise, but not unless those periods of intense play let your heart and lungs work to their fullest. If that doesn't occur—if you're just "fooling around"—the sport is probably enhancing nothing more than your coordination and flexibility.

No matter how fast-moving or exciting they are, such sports are not intended to be the keystone of your physical fitness program.

EXERCISE PROGRAM

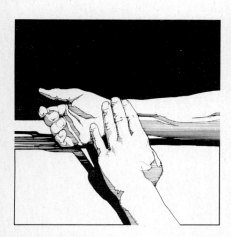

These exercises meet three basic requirements. They are designed to improve heart/lung efficiency, tone up and strengthen major muscle groups, and improve joint and body flexibility.

The exercises listed in the fitness chart on the opposite page are described individually beginning on page 33.

As you start your exercise program:

• **If you have a health problem, get your family doctor's OK.** If you're over 35, ask your doctor about the need for a stress electrocardiogram.

• **Select a regular time for exercise and stick to it.**

• **Don't try to do all of the exercises the first day of the program.** Nothing discourages a beginning exerciser like overly stiff muscles the next day. Start with a few exercises done slowly and add others gradually as your fitness improves.

• **Keep track of your progress.** The chart on page 29 will record your improvement and will help keep you motivated.

YOUR SCHEDULE

The exercises outlined on the following pages will work best for you if you follow this schedule:

Include flexibility and heart/lung exercises in your routine at least five times a week.

Strength exercises should be done only every other day (Monday, Wednesday, Friday for instance). This schedule allows your muscles time to rest and prepare for the next session.

Begin each exercise session by hopping up and down or walking briskly to increase the heart rate, warm the body, and prepare it for stretching. Then continue the routine with five or six minutes of stretching and flexibility exercises done slowly and deliberately. Do not bounce or pull in an attempt to stretch muscles. At the first sign of tension, hold for several seconds, then release and repeat.

Follow the initial stretching exercises with heart/lung and strength exercises, and always end your exercise session with a few more minutes of stretching.

HEART/LUNG GOALS

The goal of all cardio-respiratory exercise is to keep your heart beating at about 70 percent of its maximum rate for 12 to 15 minutes. The chart in the next column shows approximate ranges for maximum heartbeat and 70 percent levels. To be more precise, subtract your age from 220. That gives you the approximate maximum heart rate for your age. Then multiply by .70 to get your approximate 70 percent level.

Five minutes after you've finished your heart/lung exercise, check your pulse. If your rate is above 120, you've probably overexerted and should slow your pace the next time out.

AGE	MHR	70%
20-29	200-191	140-134
30-39	190-181	133-127
40-49	180-171	126-120
50-59	170-161	119-113
60-69	160-151	112-106

HOW TO TAKE YOUR PULSE

You'll want to check your pulse frequently, especially when you're beginning the exercise program. The best way is to find the "pulse point" on the palm side of the wrist near the thumb (see illustration). Place your second and third fingertips over the point for ten seconds and count the beats. Multiply that figure by six to get your pulse rate for one minute. You can also locate your pulse in the large arteries on either side of the neck, but applying pressure at these points may restrict the flow of blood to the brain which is dangerous at any time, but especially after exercise.

PERSONAL FITNESS CHART

FLEXIBILITY EXERCISES

EXERCISE	GOAL	WEEK 1	WEEK 2	WEEK 3	WEEK 4
Side-To-Side Bend (p.33)	5				
Forward Bend, Legs Split (p.34)	3				
Calf Stretch (p.37)	3				
Neck Roll (p.38) Clockwise	3				
Counterclockwise	3				
Alternate Toe Touch (p.41)	10				
Groin Muscle Stretch (p.42)	4 ea. leg				

HEART/LUNG EXERCISES

We've left a blank for you to fill in the name of the heart/lung exercise you choose. Your eventual goal is to keep your heart at about 70 percent of its maximum rate for 12 to 15 minutes. The chart will help you keep track of your improvement in the distance (D) you cover (or the number of repetitions if you choose jumping rope, jogging in place, or stepping up and down on a stool), the time (T) it takes you to do it, and your heart rate (HR). Remember, you won't be able to jog or jump rope for 12 to 15 minutes at first. Start slowly and exercise as long as you can at the 70 percent maximum heart rate. You probably won't see daily improvement, so the chart should be filled in at the beginning and end of each of the four weeks.

WEEK 1						WEEK 2						WEEK 3						WEEK 4					
D	T	HR	D	T	HR	D	T	HR	D	T	HR	D	T	HR	D	T	HR	D	T	HR	D	T	HR

Exercise _____

Your MHR _____

Your 70% level _____

STRENGTH EXERCISES

EXERCISE	GOAL	WEEK 1	WEEK 2	WEEK 3	WEEK 4
Squats (p.59)	10-15				
Lunge (p.60)	10 ea. leg				
Thigh Exercises Inside Thigh (p.62)	3				
Outside Thigh (p.65)	3				
Back of Thigh (p.66)	3				
Calf Exercise (p.69)	5-10				
Push-Ups (p.71)	10-15				
Chin-Ups (p.72)	5-10				
Neck Exercises (p.75) Pull Forward	1				
Forehead Push	1				
Side Push	1				
Chest Muscle Exercise (p.76)	10				
Pull-Over (p.79)	10				
Shoulder Exercises Forward Lift (p.80)	10				
Side Lift (p.83)	10				
Abdomen/Spine Exercises Back Lift (p.85)	3-5				
Sit-Ups (p.86)	15				
Leg Raises (p.88)	15 ea. leg				

PUT-IT-TOGETHER
GUIDE TO FOOD & FITNESS

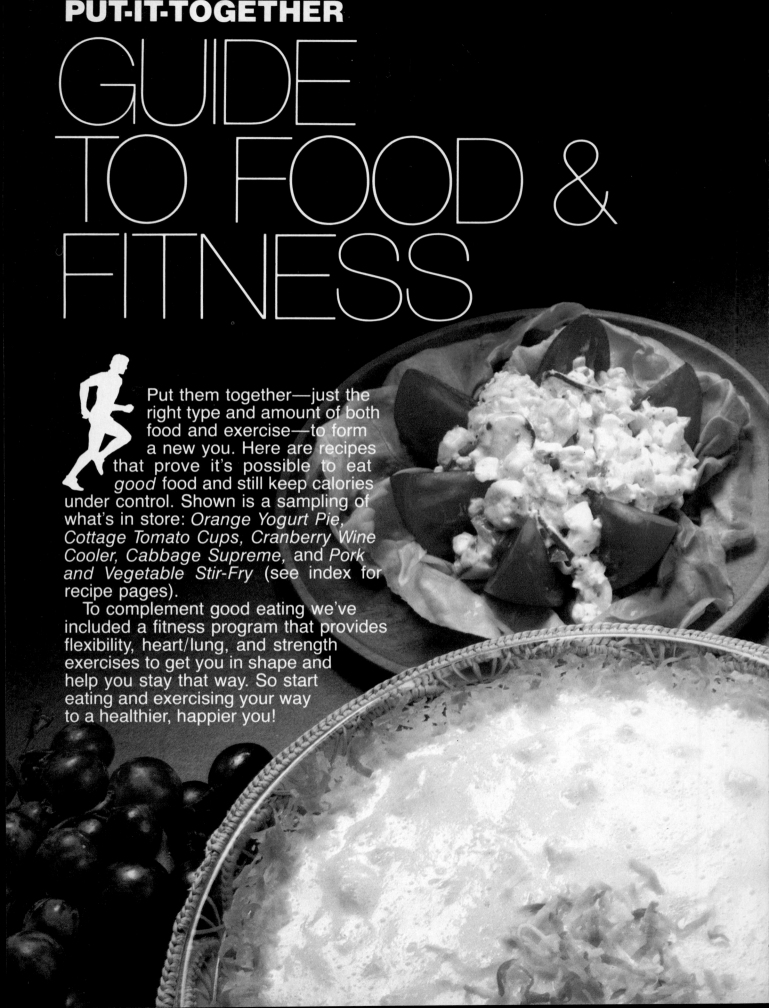

Put them together—just the right type and amount of both food and exercise—to form a new you. Here are recipes that prove it's possible to eat *good* food and still keep calories under control. Shown is a sampling of what's in store: *Orange Yogurt Pie, Cottage Tomato Cups, Cranberry Wine Cooler, Cabbage Supreme*, and *Pork and Vegetable Stir-Fry* (see index for recipe pages).

To complement good eating we've included a fitness program that provides flexibility, heart/lung, and strength exercises to get you in shape and help you stay that way. So start eating and exercising your way to a healthier, happier you!

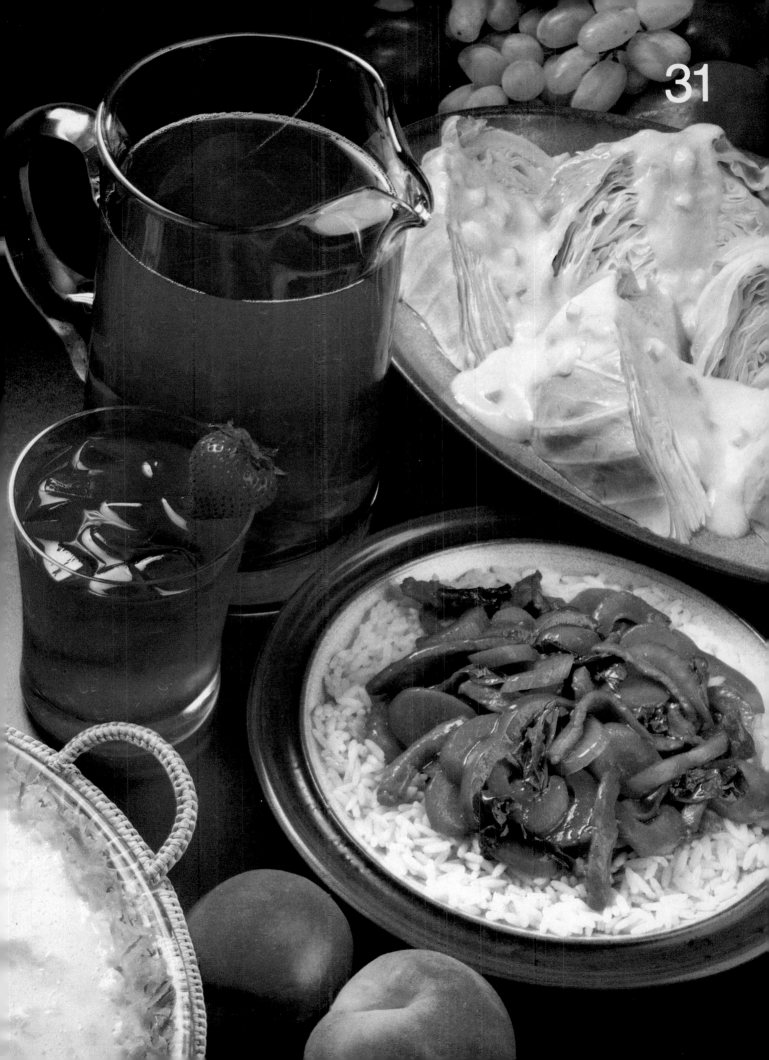

MAIN DISHES

ROAST BEEF CARBONNADE

2 **pounds lean boneless beef top round, bottom round, *or* eye round steak, cut 1½ to 2 inches thick and trimmed of fat**
Non-stick vegetable spray coating
1 **12-ounce can beer**
2 **tablespoons catsup**
1 **clove garlic, minced**
½ **teaspoon dried thyme, crushed**
1 **10-ounce package frozen brussels sprouts**
6 **medium carrots, bias sliced into ½-inch pieces (1 pound)**
2 **medium onions, cut into wedges**
2 **tablespoons cold water**
1 **tablespoon cornstarch**
¼ **teaspoon salt**
⅛ **teaspoon pepper**

Sprinkle meat with a little salt and pepper. Spray bottom of 4-quart Dutch oven with non-stick vegetable spray coating. Place over medium heat. Add meat; brown on both sides. Combine beer, catsup, garlic, and thyme; pour over meat. Cover and bake in 325° oven for 1¼ hours. Rinse brussels sprouts with warm water just to separate; add to Dutch oven along with carrots and onions. Cover and bake about 45 minutes more or till vegetables and meat are tender. Remove meat and vegetables to serving platter; keep warm. Skim fat from pan juices. To make gravy, measure 1¼ cups pan juices, adding water if necessary. Combine the 2 tablespoons water and cornstarch; stir into pan juices. Cook and stir till thickened and bubbly. Cook and stir 1 to 2 minutes more. Season gravy with salt and pepper; pass with meat and vegetables. Makes 8 servings.

BEEF-BROCCOLI STIR-FRY

Stir-frying requires a small amount of oil and constant stirring to ensure uniform cooking—

¾ **pound beef top round steak, trimmed of fat**
2 **cups broccoli flowerets**
2 **medium carrots, bias sliced**
1 **teaspoon cornstarch**
½ **teaspoon sugar**
¼ **teaspoon salt**
2 **tablespoons soy sauce**
2 **tablespoons dry sherry**
2 **tablespoons cooking oil**
1 **medium onion, cut into thin wedges**

Partially freeze beef; slice thinly across the grain into bite-size strips. Cook broccoli and carrots, covered, in boiling water 2 minutes; drain. Mix cornstarch, sugar, and salt; stir into soy sauce and sherry. Set aside.

Preheat a wok or large skillet over high heat; add 1 *tablespoon* of the oil. Stir-fry broccoli, carrots, and onion in hot oil over high heat about 3 minutes or till crisp-tender. Remove vegetables. Add the remaining 1 tablespoon oil. Add the beef to wok or skillet; stir-fry 2 to 3 minutes or till browned. Stir soy mixture; stir into beef. Cook and stir till thickened and bubbly. Stir in broccoli, carrots, and onion; cover and cook 1 minute more. Serve immediately. Makes 4 servings.

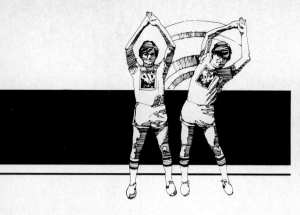

SIDE-TO-SIDE BEND
Start with arms over head, feet shoulder-width apart, and body erect. Bend laterally to the right at the waist. Hold five to ten seconds, then bend to the left and hold five to ten seconds. Repeat five times. Excellent for firming the waistline.

SAUCY PEPPER BURGERS

¼ cup fine dry bread crumbs
2 tablespoons milk
½ teaspoon dried basil, crushed
½ teaspoon dried oregano, crushed
¼ teaspoon garlic powder
¼ teaspoon salt
   Dash pepper
¾ pound lean ground beef
2 medium onions, thinly sliced
¾ cup tomato sauce
¼ cup dry red wine
2 medium green peppers, cut into strips

In a bowl combine bread crumbs, milk, basil, oregano, garlic powder, salt, and pepper. Add meat; mix well. Shape meat mixture into four ¾-inch-thick patties. In 10-inch skillet brown meat patties on both sides. Drain off fat. Add onions to skillet with meat patties. Combine tomato sauce and wine; pour over patties. Cover and simmer for 10 minutes; add green pepper strips. Cover and simmer 8 to 10 minutes more or till green pepper is just tender. Makes 4 servings.

PARED-DOWN PIZZA

This recipe makes enough dough for two pizza crusts; use one now and freeze the other for use later—

½ pound lean ground beef
1 clove garlic, minced
1 16-ounce can tomatoes, finely cut up
½ cup coarsely chopped onion
½ cup chopped green pepper
1 teaspoon dried oregano, crushed
½ teaspoon fennel seed
¼ teaspoon salt
1¾ to 2 cups all-purpose flour
1 package active dry yeast
¼ teaspoon salt
⅔ cup warm water (115° to 120°)
1 tablespoon cooking oil
   Non-stick vegetable spray coating
1 cup shredded mozzarella cheese (4 ounces)

In medium saucepan cook ground beef and garlic till meat is browned; drain well. Stir in undrained tomatoes, onion, green pepper, oregano, fennel seed, and ¼ teaspoon salt. Bring to boiling; reduce heat. Boil gently, uncovered, about 30 minutes or till of desired consistency. Meanwhile, in small mixer bowl combine ¾ cup of the flour, the yeast, and remaining ¼ teaspoon salt. Add water and oil. Beat at low speed of electric mixer ½ minute, scraping bowl constantly. Beat 3 minutes at high speed. Stir in as much of the remaining flour as you can mix in with a spoon. Turn out onto lightly floured surface. Knead in enough of the remaining flour to make a moderately stiff dough that is smooth and elastic (6 to 8 minutes total). Divide dough in half. Cover dough and let rest 10 minutes. On lightly floured surface roll each half into a 13-inch circle. Transfer circles to 12-inch pizza pans or baking sheets sprayed with non-stick vegetable spray coating. Build up edges slightly. Bake in 425° oven about 12 minutes or till lightly browned. Freeze one crust for later use. Spread remaining crust with the meat-tomato mixture. Sprinkle with mozzarella cheese. Bake for 12 to 15 minutes more or till bubbly. Makes 6 servings.

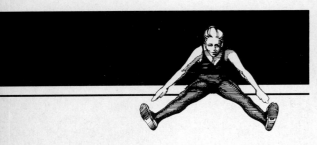

FORWARD BEND, LEGS SPLIT
Sit erect with legs apart. Bend at the waist and slide your hands as far forward as possible along your legs. Eventually you'll be able to grasp your ankles with your hands. Hold five seconds and repeat three times. Excellent for back of legs and back.

HUNGARIAN ROUND STEAK

¾ pound boneless beef round steak, trimmed of fat
2 teaspoons cooking oil
½ cup water
½ teaspoon instant beef bouillon granules
2 medium parsnips, sliced
2 medium carrots, halved and quartered
¼ cup sliced celery
2 teaspoons cornstarch
¼ teaspoon paprika
½ cup plain yogurt

Cut steak into 4 serving-size pieces. In 10-inch skillet brown meat on both sides in oil. Season with a little salt and pepper. Add water and bouillon granules to meat in skillet; cover and simmer 30 minutes. Halve any large parsnip slices. Add parsnips, carrots, and celery to meat; cover and simmer about 30 minutes more or till vegetables are tender. Remove meat and vegetables to a serving platter; keep warm.

Measure pan juices; add water if necessary to make ½ cup liquid. To make sauce, in same skillet stir cornstarch and paprika into yogurt. Stir in the ½ cup pan juices. Cook and stir till thickened and bubbly. Cook and stir 1 to 2 minutes more. Serve sauce over steak and vegetables. Makes 4 servings.

PEPPER BEEF STEW

Pork-flavored Oriental noodles can be found in the soup or foreign food section of most large supermarkets—

Non-stick vegetable spray coating
1 pound beef stew meat, trimmed of fat and cut into 1-inch cubes
1 16-ounce can tomatoes, cut up
½ cup chopped onion
1 clove garlic, minced
1 teaspoon instant beef bouillon granules
2 green peppers, cut into ¾-inch pieces
1 3-ounce package pork-flavored Oriental noodles
2 tablespoons cornstarch
1 tablespoon soy sauce
1 tablespoon cold water
1 cup bean sprouts

Spray medium saucepan with non-stick vegetable spray coating. In prepared saucepan brown the meat. Stir in *undrained* tomatoes, onion, garlic, and beef bouillon granules. Bring to boiling; reduce heat. Cover and simmer 1¼ to 1½ hours or till meat is nearly tender. Add green peppers. Simmer, covered, for 10 to 15 minutes more. Meanwhile, prepare pork-flavored noodles according to package directions; drain well. Combine cornstarch, soy sauce, and water; add to meat mixture. Cook and stir till thickened and bubbly; cook and stir 1 to 2 minutes more.

Toss together pork-flavored noodles and bean sprouts. Serve meat mixture over noodle mixture. Makes 4 servings.

Hungarian Round Steak ▶

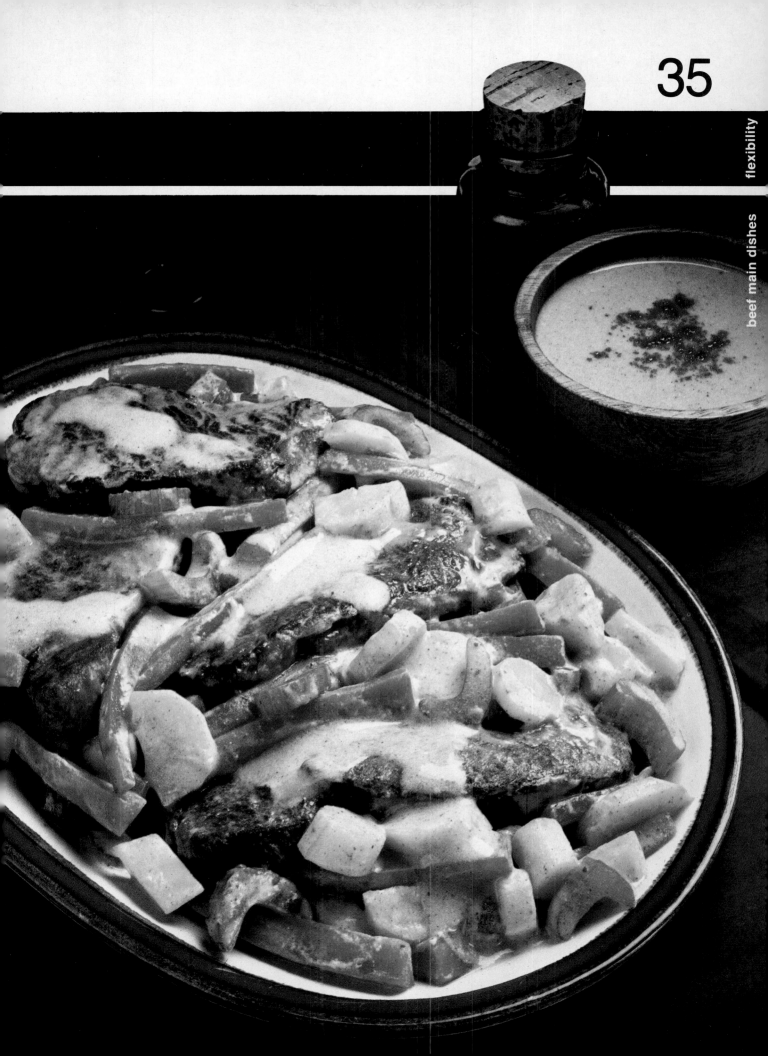

VEAL SAUTÉ WITH MUSHROOMS

¾ pound boneless veal leg round
    steak, trimmed of fat
1 tablespoon butter *or* margarine
1 teaspoon Worcestershire sauce
1 clove garlic, minced
1 medium onion, sliced and
    separated into rings
1 cup sliced fresh mushrooms
⅓ cup water
1 tablespoon lemon juice
1½ teaspoons instant beef bouillon
    granules
2 teaspoons cornstarch
2 cups hot cooked noodles
    Lemon wedges

Cut veal into 4 pieces; pound with meat mallet to ¼-inch thickness. In 10-inch skillet combine butter or margarine, Worcestershire sauce, and garlic. Cook over medium-high heat till garlic is lightly browned. Add veal and onion; cook meat on both sides till lightly browned. Arrange mushrooms over meat. Add water, lemon juice, and bouillon granules to meat and vegetables in skillet. Reduce heat; cover and simmer about 5 minutes or till meat is done. Remove meat; keep warm. Combine cornstarch and the ¼ cup *cold water*; stir into meat mixture. Cook and stir till slightly thickened and bubbly. Cook and stir 1 to 2 minutes more. Serve meat and sauce over hot noodles. Garnish with lemon wedges. Makes 4 servings.

VEAL STEW

1¼ pounds lean boneless veal, cut
    into 1-inch cubes
1 clove garlic, minced
1 tablespoon butter *or* margarine
1¾ cups water
¼ cup dry white wine
2 medium potatoes, peeled
    and cubed
2 medium carrots, bias sliced into
    1-inch pieces
½ medium onion, cut into 1-inch
    pieces
1 cup frozen peas
18 fresh mushrooms, halved
2 tablespoons snipped parsley
2 teaspoons instant chicken
    bouillon granules
½ teaspoon dried marjoram,
    crushed
2 tablespoons cold water
1 tablespoon cornstarch

In 4-quart Dutch oven cook meat and garlic in butter or margarine till meat is brown. Stir in the 1¾ cups water and the wine. Bring to boiling. Reduce heat; cover and simmer for 30 minutes. Stir in potatoes, carrots, onion, peas, mushrooms, parsley, bouillon granules, marjoram, ½ teaspoon *salt*, and ¼ teaspoon *pepper*. Cover and cook about 30 minutes more or till meat and vegetables are tender. Skim off fat. Combine the 2 tablespoons water and cornstarch; stir into meat mixture. Cook and stir till thickened and bubbly. Cook and stir 1 to 2 minutes more. Makes 6 servings.

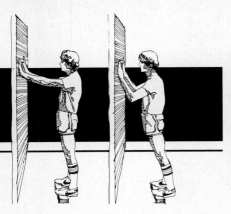

CALF STRETCH
Stand at arm's length from the wall. Place your toes on the edge of a 2x4 and your heels on the floor. Make sure the board doesn't move. Lean forward, keeping heels on the floor and body straight. You will feel stretching in the back of your lower legs. Hold the position five to ten seconds and repeat three times.

PORK AND VEGETABLE STIR-FRY   (pictured on page 31)

If you don't have a wok, a large skillet can be used to prepare this colorful stir-fry—

1	**pound lean boneless pork, trimmed of fat**
¼	**cup soy sauce**
2	**tablespoons dry sherry**
1	**tablespoon cornstarch**
¼	**teaspoon ground ginger**
2	**tablespoons cooking oil**
1½	**cups thinly bias-sliced carrots**
1½	**cups bias-sliced celery**
1	**large green pepper, cut into strips**
2	**cups torn fresh spinach leaves**
2	**cups hot cooked rice**

Partially freeze pork; slice thinly into bite-size strips. Stir together soy sauce, sherry, cornstarch, and ginger; set aside.

Preheat a wok or large skillet over high heat; add oil. Stir-fry carrots, celery, and green pepper for 2 minutes. Remove vegetables. Add another tablespoon of oil if necessary. Add the pork to wok or skillet; stir-fry for 2 to 3 minutes. Stir soy mixture; stir into pork. Cook and stir till thickened and bubbly. Stir in cooked vegetables and spinach; cover and cook for 1 minute. Serve over hot rice. Makes 6 servings.

PORK AND KRAUT SKILLET

Just 328 calories per serving in this calorie-trimmed German favorite—

	Non-stick vegetable spray coating
4	**pork top loin chops, cut ½ inch thick and trimmed of fat**
1	**8-ounce can sauerkraut, drained and rinsed**
1	**cup shredded peeled potato (1 large)**
¼	**cup chopped onion**
1	**tablespoon brown sugar**
1	**teaspoon caraway seed**
¼	**teaspoon salt**
1	**large apple, thinly sliced**
½	**cup beer**
1	**tablespoon snipped parsley**

Spray bottom of a 10-inch skillet with non-stick vegetable spray coating. Place over medium heat; brown chops on both sides. Sprinkle with a little salt and pepper; remove chops from skillet and set aside. In same skillet combine sauerkraut, shredded potato, onion, brown sugar, caraway seed, and salt; toss to mix. Arrange half of the apple slices atop sauerkraut mixture; pour beer evenly over all. Place chops atop. Cover and cook over medium heat about 20 minutes or till chops are nearly tender. Arrange remaining apple slices atop; cover and continue cooking for 5 minutes more. Garnish with snipped parsley. Serves 4.

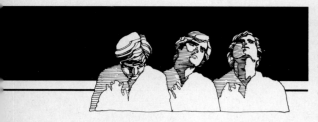

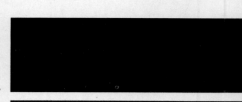

ORANGE-SPICED PORK CHOPS (pictured on page 21)

Simmer pork chops in orange juice and top with a light-flavored sauce filled with bits of fresh orange and a hint of spice. The menu on page 21 will give you an idea for putting this recipe together with other foods to make a meal—

    Non-stick vegetable spray coating
6 **pork top loin chops, cut ½ inch thick and trimmed of fat**
¼ **teaspoon salt**
⅛ **teaspoon pepper**
¼ **cup orange juice**
2 **oranges**
1 **cup water**
1 **tablespoon sugar**
1 **tablespoon cornstarch**
1 **cup orange juice**
⅛ **teaspoon ground allspice**

Spray bottom of a 12-inch skillet with non-stick vegetable spray coating; brown pork chops on both sides. Season with salt and pepper; add the ¼ cup orange juice. Cover; simmer 25 to 30 minutes or till tender.

Meanwhile, using a vegetable peeler, remove a very thin layer of the peel from one of the oranges. Slice the peel into julienne strips. Peel and section both oranges and cut sections into ½-inch pieces; set aside. Simmer orange peel strips in the water for 15 minutes; drain well and set aside.

To make sauce, in small saucepan combine sugar and cornstarch. Stir in the 1 cup orange juice. Cook and stir till thickened and bubbly. Add the orange pieces, peel, and allspice. Cook and stir 1 to 2 minutes more. Serve sauce warm over pork chops. Makes 6 servings.

PORK PAPRIKASH

Yogurt adds tang and richness, yet helps trim calories (only 263 per serving)—

1 **pound pork tenderloin, trimmed of fat and partially frozen**
    Non-stick vegetable spray coating
1 **cup chopped onion**
¾ **cup water**
2 **teaspoons paprika**
1 **teaspoon instant chicken bouillon granules**
1 **tablespoon cornstarch**
¾ **cup plain yogurt**
¼ **cup snipped parsley**
2½ **cups hot cooked noodles**

Slice pork diagonally into ¼-inch slices. Spray bottom of a 10-inch skillet with non-stick vegetable spray coating; heat skillet. In prepared skillet cook meat, half at a time, over medium-high heat about 4 minutes or till browned, stirring occasionally. Return all the meat to skillet. Add onion, water, paprika, and bouillon granules. Cover and simmer about 15 minutes or till pork is tender. Stir cornstarch into yogurt; blend some of the pan juices into yogurt mixture, stirring constantly. Return all to skillet. Cook and stir till bubbly; cook and stir 1 to 2 minutes more. Stir in parsley. Serve over hot noodles. Makes 5 servings.

SWEET AND SOUR LAMB

2 tablespoons cooking oil
1 pound lean boneless lamb, cut into thin slices
1 medium sweet red *or* green pepper, cut into strips
½ of an 8-ounce can bamboo shoots, drained
6 green onions, bias sliced into 1-inch pieces
1 8-ounce can pineapple chunks (juice pack)
2 tablespoons wine vinegar
2 tablespoons catsup
1 teaspoon instant chicken bouillon granules
¼ teaspoon salt
3 tablespoons cold water
4 teaspoons cornstarch
3 cups hot cooked rice

Preheat a 12-inch skillet over high heat; add cooking oil. Cook lamb till browned. Stir in pepper strips, bamboo shoots, and green onions. Cook and stir about 3 minutes or till crisp-tender. Drain pineapple, reserving juice. Add enough water to pineapple juice to make ¾ cup liquid. Stir pineapple liquid, pineapple chunks, vinegar, catsup, bouillon granules, and salt into lamb mixture; bring to boiling. Combine the 3 tablespoons water and cornstarch; stir into lamb mixture. Cook and stir till thickened and bubbly. Cook and stir 1 to 2 minutes more. Serve over hot rice. Makes 6 servings.

CASSOULET SOUP

1 cup dry navy beans
4 cups water
½ cup chopped onion
½ cup chopped celery
½ cup chopped carrot
2 teaspoons instant chicken bouillon granules
¼ pound boneless lamb, cut into ½-inch cubes
½ cup diced fully cooked ham
1 bay leaf
3 tablespoons dry white wine
1 teaspoon Worcestershire sauce
½ teaspoon dried basil, crushed
½ teaspoon dried oregano, crushed

Rinse beans. In large saucepan combine beans and water. Bring to boiling; reduce heat. Cover and simmer 2 minutes. Remove from heat. Cover and let stand 1 hour. (Or, soak beans in water overnight in covered pan.) Do not drain. Stir in onion, celery, carrot, and bouillon granules. Cover and simmer 30 minutes. Add lamb, ham, and bay leaf. Simmer, covered, 30 minutes longer. Remove bay leaf. Stir in wine, Worcestershire sauce, basil, and oregano. Turn mixture into 2-quart casserole. Cover and bake in 350° oven for 45 minutes. Uncover and bake for 40 to 45 minutes more, stirring occasionally. Serve in bowls. Makes 4 servings.

LAMB-STUFFED SQUASH (pictured on the cover)

This meal-in-one main dish combines meat, rice, and vegetable in each serving—

  3 **small acorn squash**
     Non-stick vegetable spray
       coating
  1 **pound lean ground lamb**
     or **lean ground beef**
  1 **clove garlic, minced**
  2 **green onions, bias sliced**
       into ½-inch pieces
 ½ **teaspoon salt**
 ¼ **teaspoon ground ginger**
 ¼ **teaspoon ground allspice**
  1 **beaten egg**
  2 **cups cooked rice**
  2 **tablespoons chopped pimiento**
 ½ **cup shredded Monterey Jack**
       cheese (2 ounces)

Cut squash in half crosswise; discard seeds. Sprinkle squash with a little salt. Place, cut side down, in 13x9x2-inch baking dish. Bake in 350° oven for 45 to 50 minutes or till tender. Meanwhile, spray a skillet with non-stick vegetable spray coating. In prepared skillet cook lamb and garlic till meat is brown; drain off fat. Stir in green onions, salt, ginger, and allspice. Remove from heat and allow the mixture to cool slightly. In large bowl combine beaten egg, rice, and pimiento; stir in meat mixture. Cut a thin slice from ends of squash so they will sit flat. Turn the squash cut side up in dish; fill with meat mixture. Cover dish with foil. Bake for 25 minutes. Uncover; top with cheese. Bake about 3 minutes more or till cheese is melted. Makes 6 servings.

PASTITSIO

  1 **cup elbow macaroni**
 ¾ **pound lean ground lamb**
 ½ **cup chopped onion**
  1 **8-ounce can tomato sauce**
 ¼ **cup grated Parmesan cheese**
 ½ **teaspoon salt**
 ½ **teaspoon dried thyme, crushed**
 ¼ **teaspoon ground cinnamon**
1½ **cups skim milk**
  3 **tablespoons all-purpose flour**
 ½ **teaspoon salt**
  2 **slightly beaten eggs**
     Ground cinnamon

Cook macaroni according to package directions; drain and set aside. In medium saucepan cook lamb and onion till meat is browned; drain well. Stir in macaroni, tomato sauce, *2 tablespoons* of the Parmesan cheese, ½ teaspoon salt, the thyme, and the ¼ teaspoon cinnamon. Spread meat mixture in a 10x6x2-inch baking dish.

For sauce, in screw-top jar combine ½ *cup* of the milk, the flour, and ½ teaspoon salt; cover and shake well. In saucepan combine remaining milk and the milk-flour mixture. Cook and stir till thickened and bubbly. Cook and stir 1 to 2 minutes more. Gradually stir about ½ cup of the sauce into beaten eggs; return to remaining sauce in saucepan, stirring rapidly. Stir in the remaining Parmesan cheese. Pour atop meat mixture in baking dish. Sprinkle with additional cinnamon. Bake, uncovered, in 375° oven 30 to 35 minutes or till a knife inserted just off-center comes out clean. Let stand 10 minutes before serving. Makes 6 servings.

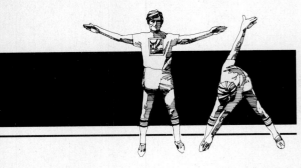

ALTERNATE TOE TOUCH
Stand erect with feet apart slightly more than shoulder width. Bend down, not twisting the body, and touch the left foot with the right hand; keep opposite hand elevated. Stand erect again, then bend and touch the right foot with the left hand. Work up to repeating the sequence ten times. Excellent for firming the waistline and stretching the hamstring muscles in your thighs.

FISH AND VEGETABLE BAKE

2 medium potatoes, peeled and cubed
1 large carrot, sliced ¼ inch thick
1 small onion, sliced ¼ inch thick
2 tablespoons butter *or* margarine, melted
1 teaspoon dried dillweed
1 teaspoon dried basil, crushed
¼ teaspoon salt
¼ teaspoon pepper
1 16-ounce package frozen fish fillets, thawed and separated
1 small green pepper, cut into rings
2 teaspoons lemon juice
1 medium tomato, coarsely chopped

In an 8x8x2-inch baking dish place potatoes, carrot, and onion. Combine melted butter or margarine, dillweed, basil, salt, and pepper; spoon half of the butter mixture atop vegetables. Cover and bake in 425° oven for 25 minutes. Place fish fillets, skin side down, atop vegetables; add green pepper rings. Combine lemon juice and remaining butter mixture; spoon over fish. Cover; bake about 15 minutes or till fish flakes easily with fork and vegetables are tender. Uncover; add chopped tomato. Return to oven; bake about 5 minutes more or till tomato is hot. Serves 4.

TUNA-CAULIFLOWER CASSEROLE

1 10-ounce package frozen cauliflower
½ cup sliced fresh mushrooms
2 tablespoons all-purpose flour
¼ teaspoon salt
1 cup evaporated skimmed milk
3 tablespoons grated Parmesan cheese
2 tablespoons sliced green onion
1 tablespoon dry white wine
1½ teaspoons lemon juice
½ teaspoon dried dillweed
Dash pepper
1 6½-ounce can tuna (water pack), drained and flaked

In saucepan cook cauliflower and mushrooms, covered, in a small amount of water for 3 minutes. Drain; cut cauliflower into small pieces. Set cauliflower and mushrooms aside. In saucepan combine flour and salt. Stir in evaporated milk. Cook and stir over low heat till thickened and bubbly. Cook and stir 1 to 2 minutes more. Remove from heat. Stir in *2 tablespoons* of the Parmesan cheese, the onion, wine, lemon juice, dillweed, and pepper. Fold in tuna, cauliflower, and mushrooms. Turn mixture into a 1-quart casserole. Sprinkle with remaining 1 tablespoon Parmesan cheese. Bake, uncovered, in 350° oven for 20 to 25 minutes or till heated through. Makes 4 servings.

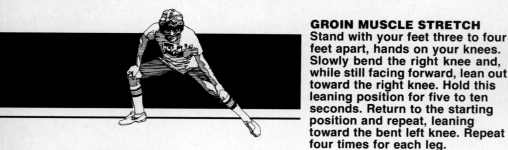

GROIN MUSCLE STRETCH
Stand with your feet three to four feet apart, hands on your knees. Slowly bend the right knee and, while still facing forward, lean out toward the right knee. Hold this leaning position for five to ten seconds. Return to the starting position and repeat, leaning toward the bent left knee. Repeat four times for each leg.

SOLE FLORENTINE

Sole is poached in a mixture of chicken broth and white wine, which is used as the base for a savory sauce—

- 1 **pound fresh *or* frozen sole fillets *or* other fish fillets**
- 1 **10-ounce package frozen leaf spinach**
- 1 **medium onion, sliced and separated into rings**
- ¼ **teaspoon salt**
- 4 **whole black peppercorns**
- ½ **cup chicken broth**
- 2 **tablespoons dry white wine**
- ½ **cup evaporated skimmed milk**
- 1 **tablespoon all-purpose flour**
- ½ **teaspoon dried dillweed**
- ¼ **teaspoon dried oregano, crushed**

Thaw fish, if frozen. Cook spinach according to package directions; drain well. Set aside and keep warm. Meanwhile, in 10-inch skillet layer fish fillets and onion. Sprinkle with salt; add peppercorns. Add chicken broth and wine; bring to boiling. Reduce heat. Cover skillet and simmer for 7 to 8 minutes or till fish flakes easily when tested with a fork. Remove fish; keep warm. Meanwhile, for sauce combine evaporated milk, flour, dillweed, and oregano; stir till smooth. Stir into mixture in skillet. Cook, stirring gently, over medium heat till thickened and bubbly. Cook and stir 1 to 2 minutes more. Remove peppercorns. Serve fish and sauce over cooked spinach. Garnish with lemon peel curls and fresh dillweed, if desired. Makes 4 servings.

TUNA-ZUCCHINI BAKE

- 5 **cups sliced zucchini**
- ½ **cup sliced fresh mushrooms**
- ¼ **cup chopped onion**
- ¼ **cup chopped green pepper**
- 1 **10¾-ounce can condensed cream of celery soup**
- 1 **tablespoon cornstarch**
- 1½ **cups dry cottage cheese**
- 1 **6½-ounce can tuna (water pack), drained and flaked**
- ¾ **teaspoon dried dillweed**
- ¼ **teaspoon garlic powder**
- ¾ **cup shredded mozzarella cheese (3 ounces)**
- 2 **tablespoons grated Parmesan cheese**
  Paprika

In large saucepan cook zucchini, mushrooms, onion, and green pepper in small amount of boiling water 4 to 5 minutes or just till crisp-tender. Drain well and set aside. In same saucepan combine soup and cornstarch; cook and stir till thickened and bubbly. Cook and stir 1 to 2 minutes more. Remove from heat. Gently stir in cottage cheese, tuna, dillweed, garlic powder, and the cooked vegetables. Turn into a 12x7½x2-inch baking dish. Sprinkle with mozzarella, Parmesan, and paprika. Bake, uncovered, in 375° oven 20 to 25 minutes or till heated through. Let stand 10 minutes before serving. Makes 8 servings.

Sole Florentine ▶

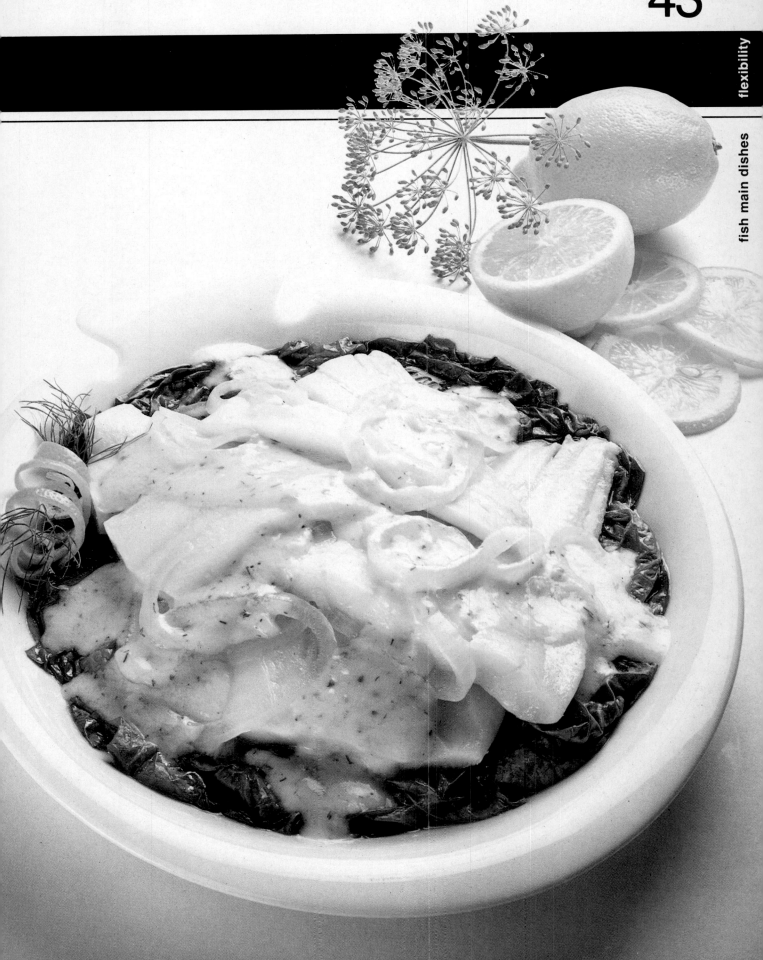

SHRIMP JAMBALAYA

½ cup chopped onion
¼ cup chopped green pepper
1 clove garlic, minced
2 tablespoons butter *or* margarine
2 tablespoons all-purpose flour
1 16-ounce can stewed tomatoes
1 cup cubed fully cooked ham
½ cup water
2 bay leaves
½ teaspoon dried thyme, crushed
¼ teaspoon salt
¼ teaspoon dried basil, crushed
¼ teaspoon ground red pepper
  Dash pepper
1 cup quick-cooking rice
1 pound frozen medium shelled
  shrimp

In saucepan cook onion, green pepper, and garlic in butter or margarine till tender. Stir in flour, blending well. Stir in *undrained* tomatoes, ham, water, bay leaves, thyme, salt, basil, red pepper, and pepper. Stir in *uncooked* rice and shrimp. Bring to boiling; reduce heat. Cover and cook over medium heat, stirring frequently, for 10 to 15 minutes or till rice and shrimp are done. Remove bay leaves. Serve in bowls. Makes 6 servings.

SESAME-SKEWERED SCALLOPS

1 pound fresh *or* frozen scallops
¼ cup dry sherry
2 tablespoons cooking oil
1 tablespoon sesame seed, toasted
  and crushed
1 teaspoon grated onion
1 clove garlic, minced
½ teaspoon salt
⅛ teaspoon pepper
1 8-ounce can pineapple chunks
  (juice pack), drained
2 medium green peppers, cut into
  1-inch pieces
12 cherry tomatoes

Thaw scallops, if frozen. Place in a plastic bag. For marinade, combine sherry, cooking oil, sesame seed, onion, garlic, salt, and pepper. Pour marinade over scallops. Close bag. Marinate in the refrigerator for several hours, turning bag occasionally. Drain, reserving marinade. Thread scallops on 6 skewers, alternating them with pineapple and green pepper. Place skewers in a 15x10x1-inch baking pan. Pour remaining marinade over skewers. Bake in 425° oven for 10 to 12 minutes or till scallops are tender, turning skewers once or twice during the cooking time. Thread tomatoes on ends of skewers. Bake 5 minutes more. Serves 6.

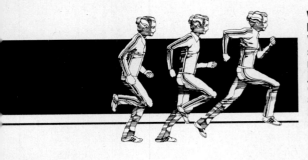

WALKING BRISKLY, RUNNING, AND JOGGING
Walking briskly produces the same benefits for your body as running and jogging—walking just takes more time. If you choose to run or jog, start by alternating 25 walking steps and 25 jogging steps. Decrease the amount of walking each day by substituting jogging steps until you're able to spend 15 minutes or more jogging.

SAVORY SAUCED CHICKEN

Chicken, especially white meat, is one of the lowest calorie choices for the main course. Remove the skin and subtract another 20 calories per serving—

1 small onion, sliced and separated into rings
1 tablespoon butter *or* margarine
1 cup vegetable juice cocktail
2 tablespoons snipped parsley
1 tablespoon cornstarch
¼ teaspoon dried marjoram, crushed
¼ teaspoon dried basil, crushed
2 whole small chicken breasts, skinned and halved lengthwise
2 tablespoons grated Parmesan cheese

In a saucepan cook onion in butter or margarine till tender but not brown. Combine vegetable juice cocktail, parsley, cornstarch, marjoram, and basil; stir into onion mixture. Cook and stir over medium heat till thickened and bubbly. Cook and stir 1 to 2 minutes more. Arrange chicken breasts in an 8x8x2-inch baking dish. Pour sauce mixture over chicken. Bake, covered with foil, in 350° oven 50 to 55 minutes or till chicken is tender. Remove foil; sprinkle with Parmesan cheese. Bake 5 to 10 minutes more. Serves 4.

CHICKEN DIVAN

Skim milk takes the place of whipping cream and mayonnaise in this calorie-reduced version of a classic main dish. Use the white meat of the chicken to lower the calorie count even more—

2 10-ounce packages frozen chopped broccoli
1⅓ cups cold water
3 tablespoons cornstarch
⅔ cup skim milk
3 tablespoons dry sherry
1½ teaspoons instant chicken bouillon granules
Dash ground nutmeg
Dash pepper
12 ounces thinly sliced cooked chicken
¼ cup grated Parmesan cheese
Paprika

Cook broccoli according to package directions; drain well. Arrange in an 8x8x2-inch baking dish. To make sauce, in a saucepan combine water and cornstarch. Stir in milk, sherry, chicken bouillon granules, nutmeg, and pepper. Cook and stir till thickened and bubbly. Cook and stir 1 to 2 minutes more. Pour *half* of the sauce over broccoli. Arrange sliced chicken atop; cover with remaining sauce. Sprinkle Parmesan cheese over sauce; sprinkle with paprika. Bake, uncovered, in 350° oven about 20 minutes or till heated through. Makes 6 servings.

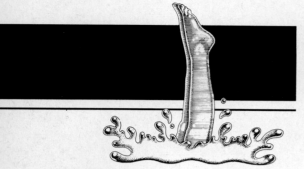

CHICKEN MARENGO

 1 3-pound broiler-fryer chicken, skinned and cut up
 1 tablespoon cooking oil
18 small boiling onions, peeled, *or* one 8-ounce can stewed onions, drained
 1 7½-ounce can tomatoes, cut up
 1 4-ounce can sliced mushrooms, drained
 ½ cup water
 ¼ cup dry sherry
 1 clove garlic, minced
 1 teaspoon instant beef bouillon granules
 2 tablespoons cold water
 1 tablespoon cornstarch

In 10-inch skillet brown chicken pieces in hot oil. Drain off excess fat. Stir in onions, *undrained* tomatoes, mushrooms, ½ cup water, sherry, garlic, and bouillon granules. Cover and cook over low heat 30 to 35 minutes or till chicken is tender. Transfer chicken, mushrooms, and onions to platter. Combine the 2 tablespoons water and cornstarch; stir into tomato mixture in skillet. Cook and stir till thickened and bubbly. Cook and stir 1 to 2 minutes more. Serve sauce over chicken. Makes 6 servings.

TURKEY-BROCCOLI PILAF

 2 cups water
 2 teaspoons instant chicken bouillon granules
 ½ cup brown rice
 ¼ cup sliced green onion
 1 small bay leaf
 1 teaspoon dried thyme, crushed
 ⅛ teaspoon pepper
 1 10-ounce package frozen cut broccoli
 ½ cup water
10 ounces cooked turkey, cut into strips (2 cups)
 2 tablespoons slivered almonds, toasted

In saucepan bring 2 cups water to boiling; add chicken bouillon granules. Stir in *uncooked* brown rice, the green onion, bay leaf, thyme, and pepper. Reduce heat; cover and simmer 45 to 50 minutes or till rice is tender. Meanwhile, cook broccoli in the ½ cup water according to package directions. *Do not drain*. Remove bay leaf. Stir turkey, almonds, and *undrained* broccoli into cooked rice mixture. Cover and simmer about 5 minutes more or till heated through. Makes 4 servings.

LEMON BROILED CHICKEN

2 whole small chicken breasts,
    skinned, halved lengthwise,
    and boned
¼ cup sliced green onion
2 tablespoons lemon juice
2 tablespoons water
2 tablespoons cooking oil
1 clove garlic, minced
½ teaspoon dried marjoram,
    crushed
½ teaspoon dried basil, crushed
¼ teaspoon dried thyme, crushed
⅛ teaspoon salt

Place each piece of chicken between two pieces of clear plastic wrap; working from center, pound with flat side of meat mallet to ¼-inch thickness. Remove plastic wrap and place chicken in plastic bag. For marinade, combine green onion, lemon juice, water, oil, garlic, marjoram, basil, thyme, and salt; pour over chicken and close bag. Marinate 30 minutes at room temperature, turning bag often. Drain, reserving marinade. Place chicken on rack of unheated broiler pan. Broil 3 to 4 inches from heat for 2 to 3 minutes, brushing often with marinade. Turn over and broil 2 to 3 minutes more, continuing to brush often with marinade. Makes 4 servings.

Meat, Fish, and Poultry: How do They Compare?

Compare the calories, protein, and fat found in similar cuts of meat to those in poultry and fish. You'll discover that meat, poultry, and fish are abundant in protein, but poultry and fish are usually lower in calories and fat.

Per Pound*	Calories	Protein (grams)	Fat (grams)
Boneless chicken (breast)	394	75	9
Walleye pike	425	88	5
Boneless veal round roast	744	89	41
Roasted turkey (light meat)	798	149	18
Boneless beef round steak	894	92	56
Lean boneless leg of lamb	1,007	81	74
Boneless pork loin roast	1,352	78	113

*all raw, except turkey (roasted)

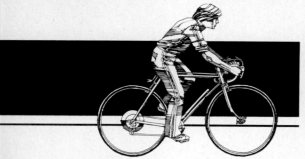

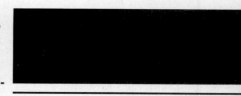

BICYCLING
Whether you ride outdoors or pedal a stationary bicycle inside, the benefits are equal. One precautionary note about bicycling: Coasting downhill and using the "easier" gears to pedal doesn't count. Use the lowest gear possible to sustain 15 minutes of riding at a pace where your heart rate is 70 percent of its maximum.

HAM AND VEGETABLE ROLL-UPS

¼ cup coarsely chopped cucumber
¼ cup coarsely chopped tomato
¼ cup sliced fresh mushrooms
2 tablespoons sliced pitted ripe olives
2 tablespoons sliced green onion
⅓ cup low-calorie Italian salad dressing
1 6-ounce package sliced fully cooked ham (8 slices)
4 large outer leaves head lettuce
1 cup shredded mozzarella cheese (4 ounces)

In a small bowl combine cucumber, tomato, mushrooms, olives, and green onion; stir in salad dressing. Cover and chill for 6 hours or overnight; drain well. To assemble roll-ups, center two ham slices atop each lettuce leaf. Top each with ¼ cup *drained* vegetable mixture and ¼ cup shredded cheese. Roll up, turning edges of lettuce in toward center while rolling; secure each roll-up with a wooden pick. Makes 4 servings.

CHICKEN 'N' SWISS STACKS

½ cup plain yogurt
3 tablespoons mayonnaise
1 tablespoon snipped parsley
1 teaspoon prepared horseradish
1 teaspoon prepared mustard
⅛ teaspoon dried rosemary, crushed
⅛ teaspoon garlic powder
1 head lettuce
2 medium green peppers, thinly sliced into rings
6 ounces Swiss cheese, sliced
6 thin slices onion
6 ounces sliced cooked chicken *or* turkey
1 medium cucumber, sliced
2 medium tomatoes, thinly sliced

Combine yogurt, mayonnaise, parsley, horseradish, mustard, rosemary, and garlic powder. Mix well; cover and chill.

Slice off core end of lettuce head. Continue cutting crosswise slices to get 6 slices that are ½ inch thick. For each stack, top lettuce slice with 2 green pepper rings, 1 ounce cheese, 1 slice onion, 1 ounce of sliced chicken or turkey, 4 cucumber slices, and 2 tomato slices. Serve each topped with 2 tablespoons of the yogurt mixture. Makes 6 servings.

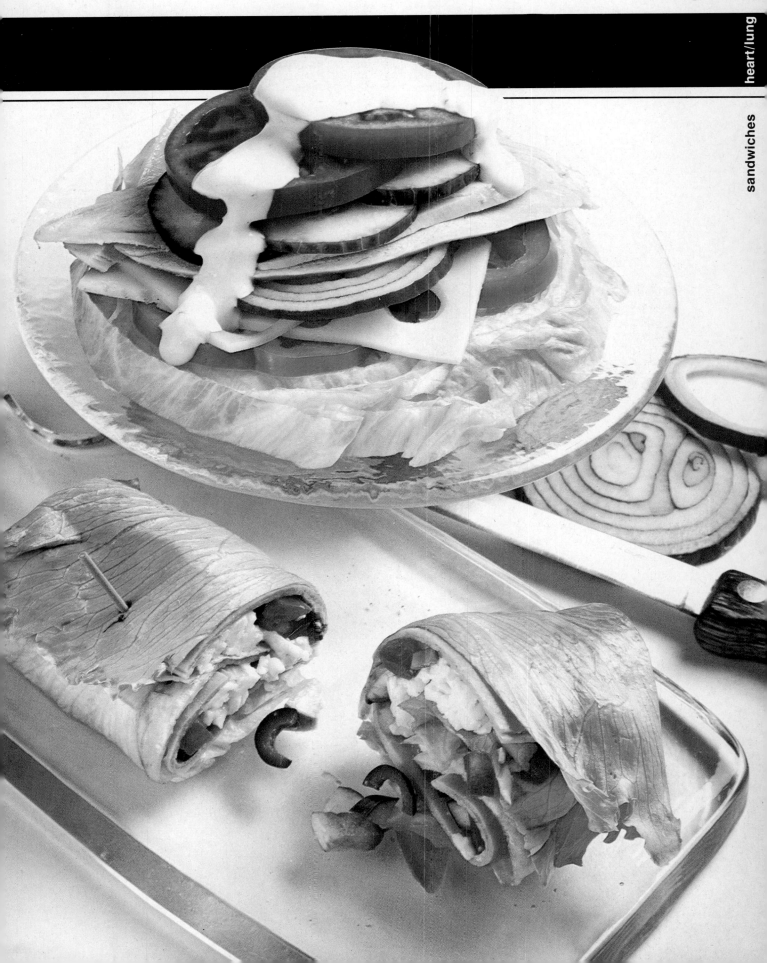

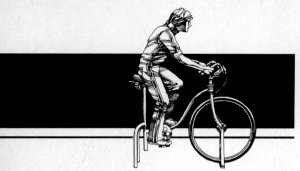

STATIONARY BICYCLE
Pedal without stopping for 12 to 15 minutes. Start with little resistance on the tire. Gradually increase the resistance as your fitness improves till you reach 65 to 70 percent of your maximum heart rate for 12 to 15 minutes.

BEEF AND SPROUT SANDWICHES

Bypassing the usual second slice of bread cuts calories in this satisfying open-face sandwich that features beef, tomatoes, and alfalfa sprouts topped with a yogurt sauce—

⅓ cup plain yogurt
2 tablespoons finely chopped cucumber
2 teaspoons snipped parsley
2 teaspoons chili sauce
4 slices rye bread, toasted
4 leaves leaf lettuce
8 ounces thinly sliced cooked beef
2 medium tomatoes, sliced (8 slices)
½ cup alfalfa sprouts

For yogurt sauce, in a small bowl combine yogurt, chopped cucumber, snipped parsley, and chili sauce.

Top each slice of toasted bread with leaf lettuce, 2 ounces sliced beef (season with salt and pepper, if desired), 2 tomato slices, 2 tablespoons alfalfa sprouts, and 2 tablespoons of the yogurt sauce. Makes 4 servings.

TUNA TACOS

Tacos are a calorie bargain when made with tuna—

2 6½-ounce cans tuna (water pack), drained and flaked
½ cup chopped celery
2 tablespoons sliced green onion
⅛ teaspoon garlic powder
5 drops bottled hot pepper sauce
¼ cup low-calorie French salad dressing *or* reduced-calorie cucumber salad dressing
12 taco shells
1½ cups chopped tomato
1½ cups shredded lettuce
¾ cup shredded cheddar cheese (3 ounces)
Taco sauce

In medium bowl combine tuna, celery, green onion, garlic powder, and hot pepper sauce; mix well. Stir in salad dressing.

Spoon tuna mixture into taco shells; top with tomato, lettuce, and cheese. Pass taco sauce. Makes 6 servings.

COOKING TO CUT CALORIES

STEAMING

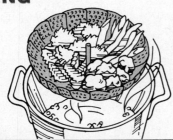

Steam cooking ensures the optimum in natural freshness and flavor because steamed foods retain their shape, texture, and nutrients. It's a popular fat-free method for cooking vegetables, and is just as suitable for meat, fish, chicken, even fruit. Although specialized appliances are available, an inexpensive metal steamer basket can be used. The metal basket is placed in a saucepan or skillet containing a shallow layer of boiling water. Food placed in the basket is cooked by steam while suspended above the boiling water in the covered saucepan or skillet.

POACHING

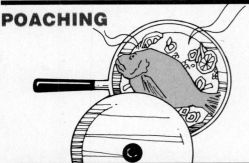

Foods traditionally sautéed and served with a rich buttery sauce can instead be poached in a fat-free liquid that doubles as the base for a delicate sauce. Poaching pans are available for fish or eggs, but standard skillets and saucepans will accommodate most cooking needs. To poach, place foods in shallow simmering liquid (broth, an inexpensive wine, or water with lemon, herbs, and spices). Cover and simmer just till done. Don't overcook. When done, fish flakes easily with a fork, chicken loses its translucency, and eggs appear set.

BROILING

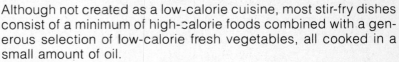

Broiling is a fast, foolproof way to hold natural flavor and juices inside foods. It's a calorie-cutting technique, too, because no added butter or oil is necessary and fats naturally present in foods are left behind in the broiler pan. Foods lacking natural oils or juices should be brushed with liquid during broiling to keep them moist. (Wine, soy sauce, and fruit juices add flavor without adding excessive calories.) For proper cooking, begin with an unheated rack in a broiler pan and broil the foods according to the time given in the recipe instructions.

STIR-FRYING

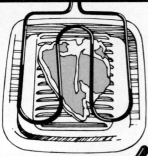

Although not created as a low-calorie cuisine, most stir-fry dishes consist of a minimum of high-calorie foods combined with a generous selection of low-calorie fresh vegetables, all cooked in a small amount of oil.

For stir-frying, cut foods in thin strips or small pieces. Then cook quickly in hot oil over high heat with constant stirring. The brief cooking time helps food retain its texture, color, and flavor. A bowl-shaped metal wok is designed for stir-frying, but a large skillet will deliver the same results.

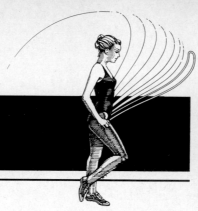

VEGETABLES

STIR-FRIED TOMATOES AND PEPPERS

1 teaspoon instant beef bouillon granules
¼ cup boiling water
2 tablespoons soy sauce
2 teaspoons cornstarch
¼ teaspoon ground ginger
  Several dashes bottled hot pepper sauce
1 tablespoon cooking oil
6 green onions, bias sliced into 1-inch pieces
½ cup bias sliced celery *or* bok choy
2 medium green peppers, cut into strips
1 cup halved cherry tomatoes

Dissolve bouillon granules in boiling water. Stir together soy sauce, cornstarch, ginger, and hot pepper sauce; stir in bouillon. Set aside.

Preheat a wok or large skillet over high heat; add cooking oil. Add green onions and celery; stir-fry 2 minutes. Remove vegetables. Add green pepper to wok or skillet; stir-fry 2 minutes. Stir soy mixture; stir into green pepper. Cook and stir till thickened and bubbly. Stir in green onions, celery, and tomatoes. Cover and cook for 1 minute. Serve immediately. Makes 6 servings.

HERBED VEGETABLE COMBO

½ pound green beans, bias sliced into 1-inch pieces (about 1½ cups)
2 small zucchini, sliced (about 2 cups)
¼ cup chopped green pepper
2 tablespoons chopped onion
2 teaspoons cooking oil
1 medium tomato, chopped
¼ teaspoon salt
¼ teaspoon dried thyme, crushed
¼ teaspoon dried rosemary, crushed
  Dash pepper

Place green beans in steamer basket. Place basket over boiling water. Cover and steam for 15 minutes. Add zucchini; cover and steam about 10 minutes more or just till vegetables are tender.

Meanwhile, in small saucepan cook green pepper and onion in hot oil till tender but not brown. Stir in tomato, salt, thyme, rosemary, and pepper. Heat through. Pour over beans and zucchini in serving bowl; toss gently. Makes 6 servings.

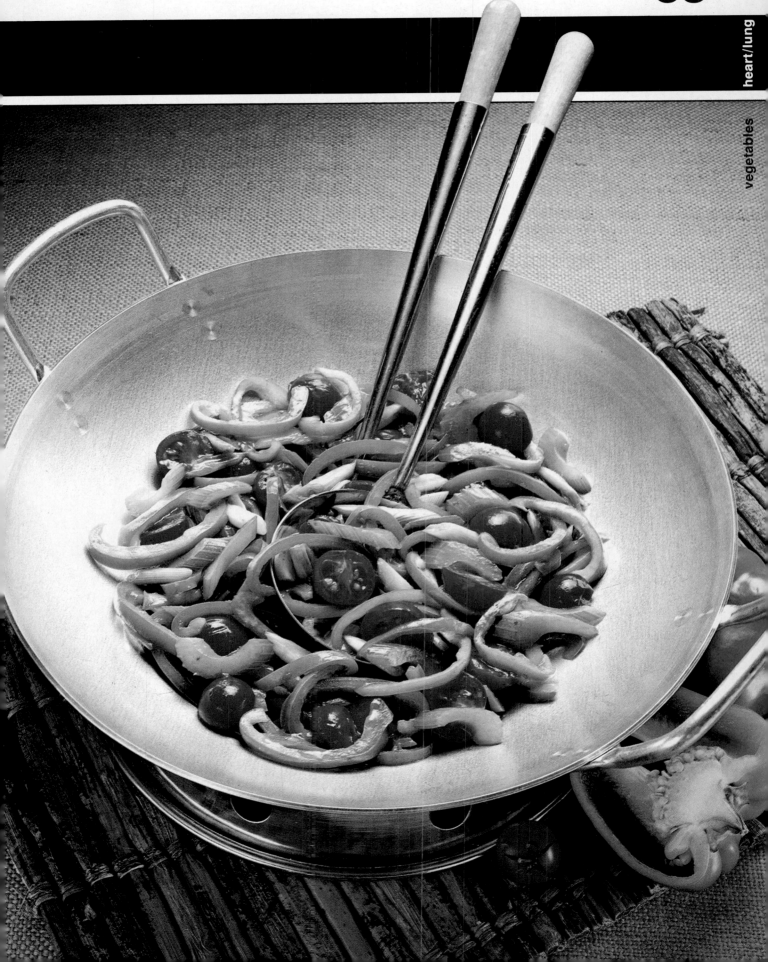

ITALIAN VEGETABLE SKILLET

¼ cup chopped onion
1 clove garlic, minced
2 tablespoons cooking oil
1 medium zucchini, sliced
1 cup frozen whole kernel corn,
    thawed
1 small green pepper, cut into
    strips
½ teaspoon dried basil, crushed
½ teaspoon dried oregano, crushed
1 small tomato, cut into wedges

In 10-inch skillet cook onion and garlic in oil till onion is tender. Stir in zucchini, corn, green pepper, basil, oregano, ¼ teaspoon *salt,* and ⅛ teaspoon *pepper.* Cook over medium heat, stirring frequently, about 5 minutes or till zucchini is crisp-tender. Stir in tomato. Cover; cook about 1 minute more or till tomato is heated through. Serve immediately. Makes 5 servings.

PARMESAN STEAMED VEGETABLES

2 cups cauliflower flowerets
    (⅓ medium head)
1 cup bias-sliced carrots
1 small green pepper, cut into
    rings
2 tablespoons butter *or* margarine
⅛ teaspoon ground nutmeg
2 tablespoons grated Parmesan
    cheese
1 tablespoon snipped parsley

Place cauliflower flowerets and carrots in steamer basket. Sprinkle with salt, if desired. Place basket over boiling water. Cover and steam for 10 minutes. Halve any large pepper rings. Add pepper rings to vegetables in basket; cover and steam for 3 to 5 minutes more or till all vegetables are tender.
  Meanwhile, in small saucepan melt butter or margarine; stir in nutmeg. Transfer vegetables to serving bowl; drizzle with melted butter mixture. Sprinkle with Parmesan cheese and parsley. Makes 6 servings.

ASPARAGUS PIQUANT

1 pound fresh asparagus, bias
    sliced into 1-inch pieces
1 small onion, thinly sliced
2 tablespoons wine vinegar
1 teaspoon sugar
¼ teaspoon mustard seed
⅛ teaspoon salt

Place asparagus and onion in steamer basket. Place basket over boiling water. Cover and steam about 10 minutes or just till vegetables are tender. Meanwhile, in small bowl combine vinegar, sugar, mustard seed, and salt.
  Transfer vegetables to a serving bowl. Pour vinegar mixture over vegetables; toss to coat. Serve immediately. Serves 4.

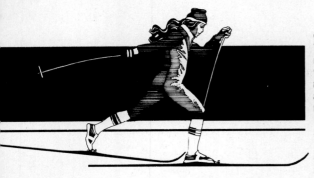

CROSS-COUNTRY SKIING
This sport provides a good work-out for your heart and lungs while you take in the scenery and crisp winter air. Start slowly and work toward mastering a rhythmic combination of swinging your arms from front to back while your legs maintain a skating motion. (Plodding along the trail wearing skis doesn't count.) It takes a little practice to develop a good gliding rhythm, so stay with it.

SESAME GREEN BEANS

½ **pound green beans** *or* **one 9-ounce package frozen French-style green beans**
1 **tablespoon butter** *or* **margarine**
2 **teaspoons sesame seed**
¼ **cup thinly sliced celery**
2 **tablespoons chopped onion**
¼ **teaspoon salt**

Slice fresh green beans diagonally end to end. In covered saucepan cook fresh beans in a small amount of boiling, lightly salted water for 10 to 12 minutes or just till tender. (*Or,* cook frozen beans according to package directions.) Drain; turn into serving bowl.

Meanwhile, in small saucepan heat butter or margarine and sesame seed over low heat about 5 minutes or till sesame seed is golden brown, stirring constantly. Add celery, onion, and salt; cook and stir till vegetables are tender. Pour over hot beans. Toss and serve immediately. Makes 4 servings.

TANGY GREEN BEANS

1 **9-ounce package frozen French-style green beans**
¼ **cup chopped onion**
2 **tablespoons snipped parsley**
1½ **teaspoons cornstarch**
¼ **teaspoon salt**
    Dash pepper
¼ **cup water**
½ **cup plain yogurt**
3 **tablespoons shredded cheddar cheese**

Cook frozen beans according to package directions along with the onion; drain.

Meanwhile, in medium saucepan combine parsley, cornstarch, salt, and pepper; stir in water. Cook and stir till thickened and bubbly. Cook and stir 1 to 2 minutes more. Stir in yogurt and bean mixture; heat through. Turn into serving dish; sprinkle with cheese. Makes 4 servings.

LEMON-GLAZED CARROTS

5 **medium carrots**
1 **tablespoon butter** *or* **margarine**
1 **tablespoon lemon juice**
⅛ **teaspoon ground nutmeg**
    Dash salt
1 **tablespoon snipped parsley**

Quarter carrots. In medium covered saucepan cook carrots in a small amount of boiling, lightly salted water 12 to 15 minutes or just till tender; drain and set aside. In same saucepan melt butter or margarine. Stir in lemon juice, nutmeg, and salt. Boil gently, uncovered, for 1 minute. Add carrots; toss gently. Turn into serving bowl; sprinkle with parsley. Makes 4 servings.

PEAS AND PODS (pictured on page 21)

2 cups shelled peas *or* one 10-ounce package frozen peas
¼ cup sliced green onion
1 6-ounce package frozen pea pods*
1 teaspoon butter *or* margarine
¼ teaspoon salt
⅛ teaspoon dried thyme, crushed
Dash pepper

Place fresh or frozen shelled peas and green onion in steamer basket. Place basket over boiling water. Cover and steam 5 minutes. Add frozen pea pods; cover and steam about 2 minutes more or till crisp-tender. Turn into serving bowl. Add butter or margarine, salt, thyme, and pepper; toss to coat. Makes 6 servings.

Note: If desired, use 6 ounces *fresh pea pods* instead of the frozen pea pods. Steam shelled peas and green onion for 3 minutes; add fresh pea pods and steam about 4 minutes more.

ORIENTAL PEA PODS AND SPINACH

1 tablespoon soy sauce
2 teaspoons lemon juice
1 teaspoon sugar
1 tablespoon cooking oil
½ teaspoon grated gingerroot
½ pound fresh small spinach leaves (6 cups)
6 ounces fresh pea pods *or* one 6-ounce package frozen pea pods

Combine soy sauce, lemon juice, and sugar; set aside. Preheat a wok or large skillet over high heat; add cooking oil. Stir-fry gingerroot in hot oil for 30 seconds. Add spinach and fresh or frozen pea pods. (If using frozen pea pods, run under cold water to separate before adding to wok; drain.) Stir-fry vegetables about 1 minute or till crisp-tender. Stir soy mixture; stir into vegetables. Heat through, tossing gently to mix. Serve immediately. Serves 6.

PEA AND CELERY MEDLEY

⅓ cup water
1½ cups frozen peas
1½ cups sliced celery
3 green onions, sliced
1 teaspoon instant chicken bouillon granules
½ teaspoon dried basil, crushed
Dash pepper
1 teaspoon butter *or* margarine

In saucepan bring water to boiling; stir in peas, celery, green onion, bouillon granules, basil, and pepper. Cover and simmer for 6 to 8 minutes or just till vegetables are tender. Drain; stir in butter or margarine. Makes 6 servings.

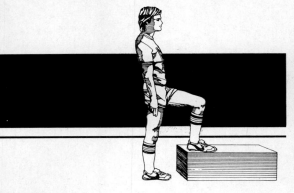

STEP-UPS
Use a small step stool or the nearest stairway. Start by putting your left foot on the stool (or step), then bring your right foot up. Next, return the left foot to the floor, then the right foot. The object is to get a steady 1-2-3-4 rhythm established. Remember to start slowly and increase gradually. An excellent 15-minute exercise for a rainy day or when you're away from home.

CHIVE CREAMED CORN

1 **10-ounce package frozen whole kernel corn**
¼ **cup chopped onion**
2 **teaspoons butter *or* margarine**
½ **cup skim milk**
1½ **teaspoons cornstarch**
¼ **teaspoon dried marjoram, crushed**
1 **ounce Neufchâtel cheese**
1 **tablespoon snipped chives**

Cook corn according to package directions; drain well. Meanwhile, in medium saucepan cook onion in butter or margarine till tender. In screw-top jar combine skim milk, cornstarch, marjoram, ¼ teaspoon *salt,* and dash *pepper;* cover and shake well. Add to onion. Cook and stir till thickened and bubbly. Cook and stir 1 to 2 minutes more. Stir in Neufchâtel cheese and chives till cheese is blended. Stir corn into cheese mixture; heat through. Serves 4.

CREAMY CORN AND ZUCCHINI (pictured on page 61)

4 **fresh ears of corn *or* one 10-ounce package frozen whole kernel corn**
2 **medium zucchini, sliced**
½ **cup cream-style cottage cheese**
¼ **cup dairy sour cream**
2 **tablespoons grated Parmesan cheese**

Cut fresh corn off cob. In covered saucepan cook fresh or frozen corn and zucchini in a small amount of boiling, lightly salted water for 3 to 5 minutes or just till tender. Drain. Combine cottage cheese, sour cream, Parmesan, ⅛ teaspoon *salt,* and ⅛ teaspoon *pepper.* Pour over hot cooked vegetables and stir gently to combine; heat through. Makes 6 servings.

SPINACH PIE

1 **10-ounce package frozen chopped spinach**
½ **cup chopped onion**
2 **cloves garlic, minced**
1 **tablespoon butter *or* margarine**
6 **beaten eggs**
⅓ **cup skim milk**
1 **cup shredded mozzarella cheese**
½ **teaspoon dried marjoram, crushed**
¼ **teaspoon dried basil, crushed**
Non-stick vegetable spray coating
¼ **cup wheat germ**

Thaw spinach; drain well. In saucepan cook onion and garlic in butter or margarine till onion is tender but not brown. Set aside.
In large bowl combine eggs and milk. Stir in the well-drained spinach, ⅔ *cup* of the cheese, the marjoram, basil, ¼ teaspoon *salt,* and ¼ teaspoon *pepper.* Stir in cooked onion and garlic. Spray a 9-inch pie plate or shallow 9-inch quiche dish with non-stick vegetable spray coating. Sprinkle wheat germ over bottom and up sides of the pie plate. Turn spinach-egg mixture into pie plate. Bake, uncovered, in 350° oven for 25 to 30 minutes or till knife inserted off-center comes out clean. Sprinkle with remaining cheese. Bake about 3 minutes more or till cheese is melted. Cut into wedges to serve. Makes 6 servings.

CHEESE-BROCCOLI BAKE

Neufchâtel cheese adds a flavor and richness similar to cream cheese with only two-thirds the calories—

½ **pound broccoli** *or* **one 10-ounce package frozen cut broccoli**
1 **cup frozen small whole onions**
1 **tablespoon cornstarch**
⅛ **teaspoon salt**
  Dash pepper
⅔ **cup skim milk**
2 **ounces Neufchâtel cheese**
2 **tablespoons grated Parmesan cheese**

Cut fresh broccoli stalks lengthwise into uniform spears, following the branching lines. Cut off buds and set aside. Cut the remaining part of spears into 1-inch pieces.

In medium covered saucepan cook the 1-inch fresh broccoli pieces in boiling, lightly salted water for 10 to 12 minutes or just till tender, adding the reserved broccoli buds for the last 5 minutes of the cooking time. (*Or,* cook the frozen broccoli according to package directions.) Drain well. Cook the frozen onions according to package directions; drain well.

In small saucepan combine cornstarch, salt, and pepper; stir in skim milk. Cook and stir till thickened and bubbly. Cook and stir 1 to 2 minutes more. Reduce heat; stir in Neufchâtel cheese till smooth.

Combine broccoli, onions, and milk mixture; stir gently to mix. Turn into 1-quart casserole. Sprinkle with Parmesan cheese. Bake, uncovered, in 350° oven for 20 to 25 minutes or till heated through. Makes 6 servings.

BAKED LIMA BEANS WITH TOMATOES

Tomatoes with a savory blend of herbs make lima beans unusually good—

1 **16-ounce can lima beans, drained**
1 **8-ounce can stewed tomatoes, cut up**
2 **tablespoons finely chopped onion**
1 **small clove garlic, minced**
¼ **teaspoon dried basil, crushed**
¼ **teaspoon dried marjoram, crushed**
¼ **cup shredded Swiss cheese (1 ounce)**

Combine lima beans, *undrained* tomatoes, onion, garlic, basil, marjoram, and dash *pepper*. Turn into a 1-quart casserole. Bake, uncovered, in 350° oven for 30 minutes. Sprinkle with cheese. Serve in sauce dishes. Makes 5 servings.

SQUATS

This is a good exercise for the front of the thighs. Begin by standing with your arms extended in front of you. Squat *slowly* until your thighs are parallel to the floor, or until your buttocks almost touch the seat of a chair. *Slowly* rise again until you are standing. Goal: 15 for men, ten for women.

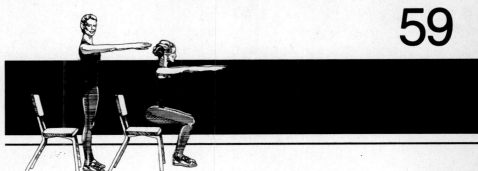

COMPANY CABBAGE

2　**teaspoons instant chicken bouillon granules**
4　**cups coarsely shredded cabbage**
½　**cup coarsely shredded carrot**
¼　**cup sliced green onion**
½　**teaspoon dillseed**
3　**tablespoons chopped pecans**
1　**tablespoon butter *or* margarine, melted**
½　**teaspoon prepared mustard**

In a large saucepan heat chicken bouillon granules in ⅓ cup *water* till dissolved. Add cabbage, carrot, green onion, dillseed, and ⅛ teaspoon *pepper.* Toss to mix. Cook, covered, over medium heat about 5 minutes or till tender, stirring once during cooking. Stir together pecans, butter or margarine, and mustard. Pour over vegetables; toss to mix. Makes 6 servings.

CABBAGE SUPREME　(pictured on page 31)

1　**medium head cabbage, cored and cut into 8 wedges**
¼　**cup chopped green pepper**
¼　**cup finely chopped onion**
1　**tablespoon butter *or* margarine**
1　**tablespoon cornstarch**
1　**cup skim milk**
⅓　**cup plain yogurt**
¼　**cup shredded cheddar cheese (1 ounce)**

In large skillet cook cabbage in a small amount of boiling, lightly salted water for 3 minutes; cover pan and cook 10 to 12 minutes more or just till tender. Drain well; place on serving platter and keep warm. Meanwhile, in saucepan cook green pepper and onion in butter or margarine till tender; add cornstarch and mix well. Stir in skim milk, ¼ teaspoon *salt,* and dash black or white *pepper.* Cook and stir till thickened and bubbly. Cook and stir 1 to 2 minutes more. Stir in yogurt and cheese till cheese melts. Pour over cabbage to serve. Makes 8 servings.

HERBED BRUSSELS SPROUTS

¾　**pound brussels sprouts**
1　**small onion, cut into thin wedges**
1　**clove garlic, minced**
1　**tablespoon butter *or* margarine**
¼　**teaspoon dried thyme, crushed**
⅛　**teaspoon salt**
⅛　**teaspoon dried oregano, crushed**
　Dash pepper

Place brussels sprouts and onion in steamer basket. Place basket over boiling water. Cover and steam about 20 minutes or till vegetables are tender.

In 10-inch skillet cook garlic in butter or margarine till lightly browned. Stir in brussels sprouts, onion, thyme, salt, oregano, and pepper. Cook for 3 to 5 minutes or till vegetables are heated through, stirring occasionally. Makes 4 servings.

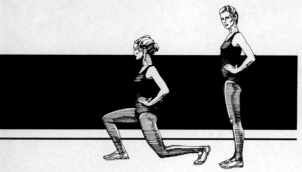

LUNGE
Start in a standing position with your hands on your hips. Lunge forward onto the right leg and slowly return to the starting position. Then lunge forward onto the left leg and return to starting position again. Goal: ten repetitions for each leg. This is another good exercise for the front of the thighs.

CURRIED POTATOES

1 pound new potatoes, halved
1 small onion, sliced
1 clove garlic, minced
¼ teaspoon curry powder
2 tablespoons butter *or* margarine
1 tablespoon snipped parsley
1 teaspoon lemon juice
¼ teaspoon salt
　Dash ground red pepper

In medium covered saucepan cook *unpeeled* potatoes and sliced onion in boiling, lightly salted water about 15 minutes or till potatoes are just tender; drain.

　Meanwhile, in small saucepan cook garlic with curry powder in butter or margarine about 1 minute. Stir in parsley, lemon juice, salt, and red pepper. Add butter mixture to potatoes and onion; toss gently to mix. Makes 4 servings.

WHIPPED POTATO BAKE

4 medium potatoes, peeled and cubed
4 ounces Neufchâtel cheese
2 tablespoons snipped chives
½ teaspoon salt
¼ teaspoon dried basil, crushed
⅛ teaspoon pepper
⅓ cup plain yogurt
2 tablespoons grated Parmesan cheese

In covered saucepan cook potatoes in boiling, lightly salted water for 10 to 15 minutes or till tender; drain. In mixing bowl combine hot potatoes, Neufchâtel cheese, chives, salt, basil, and pepper. Add yogurt; beat with electric mixer till smooth and fluffy. Turn into 1-quart casserole. Sprinkle with Parmesan cheese. Bake, uncovered, in 350° oven about 25 minutes. Makes 6 servings.

SPRINGTIME POTATOES

1 pound tiny new potatoes
½ cup chopped seeded cucumber
¼ cup sliced green onion
¼ cup sliced radishes
¼ teaspoon salt
⅛ teaspoon celery seed
　Dash pepper
½ cup plain yogurt

In covered saucepan cook *unpeeled* potatoes in boiling, lightly salted water about 15 minutes or till potatoes are just tender; drain. Halve any large potatoes. In small saucepan combine cucumber, green onion, radishes, salt, celery seed, and pepper; stir in yogurt. Cook over low heat till heated through, stirring constantly. (*Do not boil.*) Pour yogurt mixture over hot potatoes. Makes 4 servings.

Creamy Corn and Zucchini (see recipe, page 57), Curried Potatoes ▶

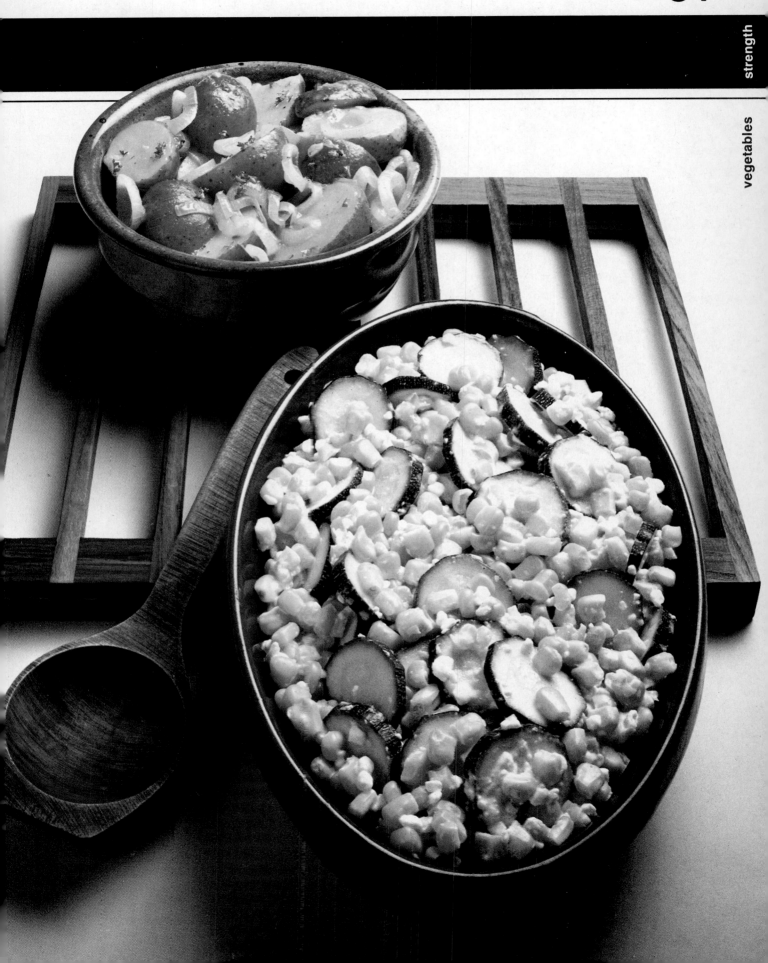

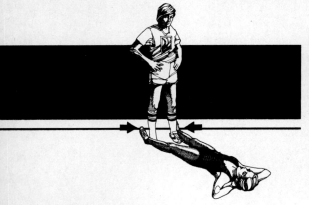

INSIDE THIGH EXERCISE
Lie on your back on the floor with feet spread two or three feet apart. Have a helper stand between your legs with ankles touching yours, or use the legs of a sturdy chair. Then try to bring your legs together. Keep the pressure on for ten seconds. Goal: three repetitions. Breathe normally two or three times during each of the ten-second repetitions.

BRANDIED SWEET POTATOES

3 medium sweet potatoes
  (1 pound)
1 11-ounce can mandarin orange
  sections
2 tablespoons brandy
1 teaspoon butter *or* margarine
⅛ teaspoon salt
⅛ teaspoon ground cinnamon
  Dash ground ginger

In medium covered saucepan cook sweet potatoes in boiling, lightly salted water for 30 to 40 minutes or till tender; drain. Peel and cut crosswise into thick pieces. Drain mandarin oranges, reserving 3 tablespoons liquid. In 10-inch skillet combine the reserved orange liquid, the brandy, butter or margarine, salt, cinnamon, and ginger. Add sweet potatoes. Cook over medium heat about 5 minutes or till potatoes are heated through and some of the liquid has evaporated, stirring in mandarin orange sections the last 1 minute of cooking. Makes 4 servings.

ZUCCHINI-STUFFED GREEN PEPPERS

4 medium green peppers
2 teaspoons butter *or* margarine
2 cups chopped zucchini
1 cup sliced fresh mushrooms
¼ cup chopped onion
1 clove garlic, minced
½ teaspoon dried basil, crushed
¼ teaspoon salt
  Dash pepper
⅓ cup plain croutons

Cut tops off green peppers; remove seeds and membrane. Precook peppers in boiling, lightly salted water about 5 minutes; drain. (*Or,* for crisp peppers omit precooking.) Sprinkle inside of peppers with a little salt. In a medium skillet melt butter or margarine; stir in zucchini, mushrooms, onion, garlic, basil, salt, and pepper. Cook, uncovered, over medium-high heat for 10 to 15 minutes or till liquid has evaporated, stirring occasionally. Stir in croutons; spoon mixture into peppers. Place in 1½-quart casserole. Bake, covered, in 350° oven for 15 minutes; uncover and bake about 10 minutes more. Makes 4 servings.

DILLED ZUCCHINI

3 medium zucchini, sliced ⅜ inch
  thick (1 pound)
¼ cup chopped onion
1 tablespoon butter *or* margarine
1 tablespoon snipped parsley
1 teaspoon lemon juice
¼ teaspoon dried dillweed

In covered saucepan cook zucchini and onion in small amount of boiling, lightly salted water about 5 minutes or just till tender. Drain well. Add butter or margarine, parsley, lemon juice, and dillweed; sprinkle with a little salt and pepper. Toss to coat. Makes 4 servings.

CRUSTLESS VEGETABLE QUICHE

A rich, creamy quiche with only 75 calories per serving—

¾ **pound spinach**
⅔ **cup thinly sliced green onion**
1 **cup chopped lettuce**
¼ **cup snipped parsley**
3 **eggs**
⅓ **cup plain yogurt**
2 **ounces Neufchâtel cheese,**
    softened
¼ **cup skim milk**
⅛ **teaspoon pepper**
    Dash salt
    Dash Worcestershire sauce
1 **tablespoon grated Parmesan**
    cheese

Rinse and chop spinach, removing stems. Cook spinach and onion, covered, with just the water that clings to spinach till steam forms. Reduce heat and cook 3 to 5 minutes, turning spinach frequently. Drain. Stir in lettuce and parsley. With electric mixer beat together eggs, yogurt, Neufchâtel cheese, milk, pepper, salt, and Worcestershire till smooth. Stir in spinach mixture. Turn into a greased 9-inch pie plate; sprinkle with Parmesan cheese. Bake, uncovered, in 375° oven for 25 to 30 minutes or till knife inserted just off-center comes out clean. Let stand 10 minutes before serving. Makes 8 servings.

ZUCCHINI OREGANO

Dry white wine adds an elegant flavor to zucchini—

4 **small zucchini, sliced (1 pound)**
4 **green onions, bias sliced into**
    ½-inch pieces
2 **tablespoons dry white wine**
1 **teaspoon lemon juice**
1 **teaspoon butter *or* margarine**
½ **teaspoon dried oregano, crushed**
⅛ **teaspoon salt**
    Dash pepper
2 **small tomatoes, cut into thin**
    wedges
1 **tablespoon snipped parsley**

In 10-inch skillet combine zucchini, green onions, wine, lemon juice, butter or margarine, oregano, salt, and pepper. Cook, uncovered, over medium-high heat about 5 minutes or till zucchini is crisp-tender and some of the liquid has evaporated, stirring occasionally. Stir in tomato wedges and parsley. Cover and cook for 1 minute. Makes 6 servings.

SPICED BEETS AND APPLE

Apples, orange juice, and a hint of spice give beets a change of pace—

¾ pound beets *or* one 16-ounce
    can sliced beets, drained
1 medium apple, peeled, cored,
    and sliced
¼ cup chopped onion
2 teaspoons butter *or* margarine
1 teaspoon sugar
1 teaspoon lemon juice
¼ teaspoon ground allspice
⅛ teaspoon salt
    Dash pepper
½ cup orange juice
1½ teaspoons cornstarch

Peel and slice fresh beets. In medium covered saucepan cook fresh beets in small amount of boiling, lightly salted water for 15 to 20 minutes or just till tender; drain.

In same saucepan cook apple and onion in butter or margarine till tender. Stir in fresh or canned beets, sugar, lemon juice, allspice, salt, and pepper. Combine orange juice and cornstarch; add to saucepan. Cook and stir till thickened and bubbly. Cook and stir 1 to 2 minutes more. Makes 4 servings.

FRESH PEA SOUP

This soup has a flavor and texture reminiscent of a rich cream soup, minus many of the calories—

2 cups shelled peas *or* one 10-
    ounce package frozen peas
3 ounces spinach (about 7 leaves)
2 ounces lettuce (about 10 leaves)
½ cup chopped leeks
2 teaspoons instant chicken
    bouillon granules
½ teaspoon dried chervil, crushed
⅛ teaspoon pepper
1¼ cups water
¾ cup skim milk
2 teaspoons butter *or* margarine

In large saucepan combine peas, spinach, lettuce, leeks, bouillon granules, chervil, and pepper; add water. Bring to boiling; reduce heat. Cover and simmer for 20 minutes. Pour into blender container or food processor bowl; cover and process till smooth. Sieve mixture back into pan. Add milk and butter or margarine; heat through. Makes 4 servings.

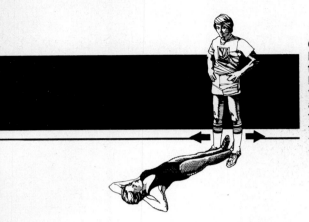
OUTSIDE THIGH EXERCISE
Lie on your back on the floor with feet about a foot apart. Have a helper stand with legs outside of yours. Try to spread your legs apart. Keep the pressure on for ten seconds. Goal: three repetitions. Breathe normally two or three times during each of the ten-second repetitions.

BROCCOLI-CAULIFLOWER SOUP

1 10-ounce package frozen chopped broccoli
1 10-ounce package frozen cauliflower
⅓ cup chopped onion
2 teaspoons instant chicken bouillon granules
1½ cups water
¼ teaspoon ground mace
3 cups skim milk
1 tablespoon cornstarch
¼ cup shredded *process* Swiss cheese (1 ounce)

In large saucepan cook frozen broccoli and cauliflower with onion and chicken bouillon granules in the 1½ cups water for 5 to 8 minutes or till vegetables are tender. *Do not drain.* In blender container blend *half* of the vegetable mixture at a time and the mace till smooth. Return all blended vegetables to saucepan. Combine ½ *cup* of the milk and the cornstarch; add to vegetable mixture. Stir in the remaining milk, ½ teaspoon *salt,* and dash *pepper.* Cook and stir till thickened and bubbly. Cook and stir 1 to 2 minutes more. Add shredded cheese; stir till melted. Makes 8 servings.

CHILLED SPINACH BISQUE

1 10-ounce package frozen chopped spinach
2 cups water
¼ cup sliced green onion
1 tablespoon instant chicken bouillon granules
⅛ teaspoon ground nutmeg
4 ounces Neufchâtel cheese, cubed
Lemon twists

In saucepan combine spinach, water, green onion, instant chicken bouillon granules, and nutmeg. Cover and simmer about 5 minutes or till vegetables are tender. *Do not drain.* Add Neufchâtel cheese. Pour *half* the spinach mixture at a time into blender container or food processor bowl; cover and blend till smooth. Pour into a bowl; cover and chill. Garnish with lemon twists. Makes 4 servings.

CHILLED ASPARAGUS SOUP

1 pound fresh asparagus, cut up, *or* one 10-ounce package frozen cut asparagus
¼ cup chopped onion
2 cups skim milk
½ teaspoon salt
Dash white pepper

Cook fresh asparagus and onion, covered, in small amount of boiling, lightly salted water for 6 to 8 minutes or just till tender. (*Or,* cook frozen asparagus according to package directions along with the onion.) Drain well. In blender container combine the drained asparagus-onion mixture, ½ cup of the milk, the salt, and pepper. Cover and blend about 15 seconds or till smooth. Add remaining milk; cover and blend to mix. Cover and chill at least 3 hours or overnight (chill in blender container, if desired). Stir or blend before serving. Makes 6 servings.

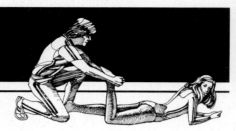

BACK OF THIGH EXERCISE
Lie on the floor on your stomach.
Bend your right knee about 90
degrees. Have a helper hold your
ankle. Then *try* to move your leg
to your back and keep trying for
ten seconds. Goal: three repetitions for each leg.

SALADS

SPICED FRUIT MOLD

  1 cup apple juice *or* apple cider
  4 inches stick cinnamon
  4 whole cloves
  1 envelope unflavored gelatin
  ¾ cup orange juice
  1 cup chopped apple (1 medium)
  ⅔ cup orange sections, chopped
    (2 medium)

In saucepan combine ¾ *cup* of the apple juice or cider, the cinnamon, and cloves. Simmer, covered, for 15 minutes; remove spices. Meanwhile, soften gelatin in the remaining ¼ cup apple juice or cider. Add to apple juice in saucepan; cook and stir over low heat till dissolved. Stir in orange juice. Chill till partially set (consistency of unbeaten egg whites). Fold apple and orange sections into gelatin mixture. Turn into 3½-cup mold. Chill several hours or till firm. Unmold to serve. Makes 6 servings.

CREAMY STRAWBERRY MOLD

  2 cups fresh strawberries
  1 4-serving envelope low-calorie
    strawberry-flavored gelatin
  1 cup boiling water
  ⅓ cup dairy sour cream
  ¼ cup cold water
  ½ teaspoon vanilla

In blender container or food processor bowl, puree *1 cup* of the strawberries. Slice the remaining berries; set aside. Dissolve gelatin in boiling water. Stir in pureed berries, sour cream, cold water, and vanilla. Chill till partially set (consistency of unbeaten egg whites). Beat at high speed of electric mixer till light and fluffy. Fold in remaining sliced berries. Turn into 4-cup mold. Chill several hours or till firm. Unmold to serve. Makes 6 servings.

CRANBERRY ORANGE MOLD

  1 cup fresh *or* frozen cranberries
  2 tablespoons sugar
  1 envelope unflavored gelatin
  2 cups low-calorie cranberry juice
    cocktail
  2 medium oranges, peeled,
    sectioned, and chopped

Using food processor or coarse blade of food grinder, grind cranberries. In bowl stir together cranberries and sugar; set aside. In saucepan soften gelatin in *1 cup* of the cranberry juice cocktail. Cook and stir over low heat till gelatin is dissolved. Cool. Stir in remaining 1 cup cranberry juice cocktail; chill till partially set (consistency of unbeaten egg whites). Fold cranberry mixture and chopped oranges into partially set gelatin mixture; pour into 3½-cup mold. Chill several hours or till firm. Unmold to serve. Makes 6 servings.

Spiced Fruit Mold, Zucchini Salad (see recipe, page 76) ▶

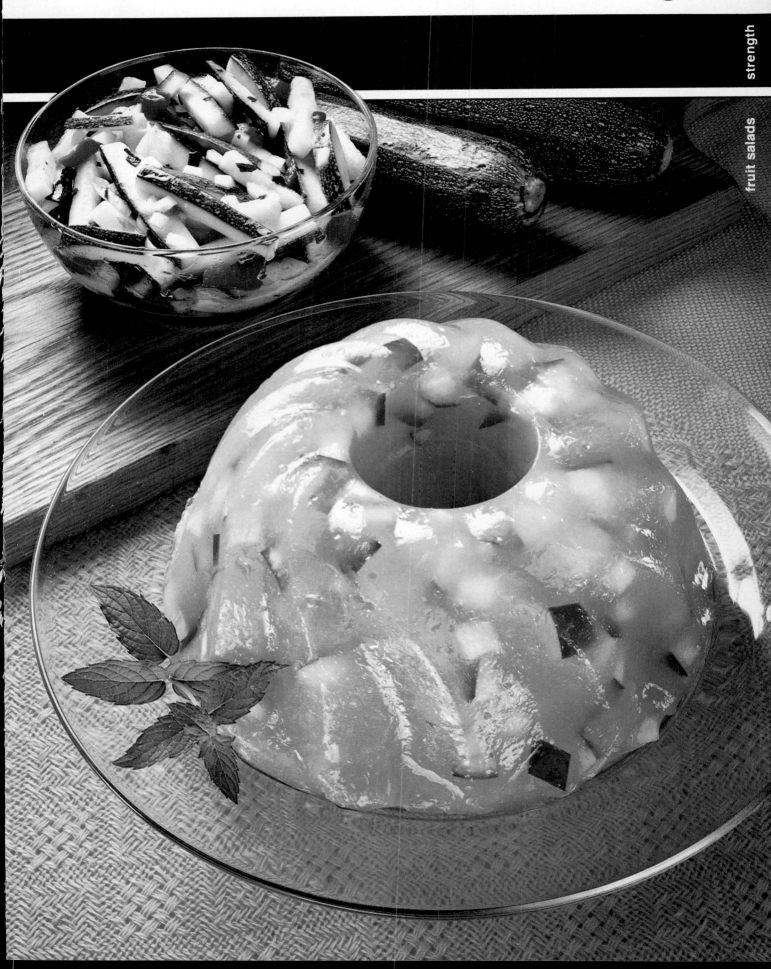

SPARKLING CHERRY-BERRY MOLD

1 envelope unflavored gelatin
¼ cup water
2 tablespoons lemon juice
1 tablespoon sugar
1 12-ounce can low-calorie
   strawberry carbonated
   beverage
½ cup pitted, halved, fresh *or*
   frozen dark sweet cherries
½ cup sliced fresh *or* frozen
   strawberries

In a small saucepan soften gelatin in water. Cook and stir over low heat till gelatin is dissolved. Add lemon juice and sugar; stir till sugar is dissolved. Stir in carbonated beverage; chill till partially set (consistency of unbeaten egg whites). Fold in cherries and strawberries. Pour into 3-cup mold. Chill several hours or till firm. Unmold to serve. Makes 4 servings.

RAINBOW FRUIT SALAD

½ medium cantaloupe, peeled and
   cubed (2 cups)
1 cup halved fresh strawberries
1 cup halved seedless green
   grapes
1 medium apple, chopped
½ cup evaporated skimmed milk,
   chilled
½ of a 6-ounce can frozen orange
   juice concentrate, partially
   thawed (⅓ cup)
6 lettuce leaves

Combine cantaloupe, strawberries, grapes, and apple; toss to mix. Combine evaporated skimmed milk and orange juice concentrate; pour over fruit and toss to coat. Serve on individual lettuce-lined plates. Makes 6 servings.

APPLE BANANA FROST

⅓ cup evaporated skimmed milk
1 cup unsweetened applesauce
1 medium banana, mashed
1 medium orange, peeled,
   sectioned, and chopped
2 tablespoons honey
8 leaves leaf lettuce

Pour milk into small mixer bowl. Place in freezer till ice crystals just begin to form around edges. Beat with electric mixer till fluffy. In another bowl combine applesauce, banana, orange, and honey. Fold whipped milk into fruit mixture. Turn into muffin pan lined with paper bake cups; freeze till firm. To serve, remove paper bake cups and invert on lettuce leaves. Let stand 5 minutes before serving. Makes 8 servings.

CALF EXERCISE
Stand with the balls of your feet on the edge of a stairstep. Balance yourself with your hand on the stair rail, then raise and lower your body on your toes to get the fullest range of motion. You can make this exercise harder by doing it one leg at a time. Goal: five to ten repetitions. This is a good exercise for building and stretching calf muscles.

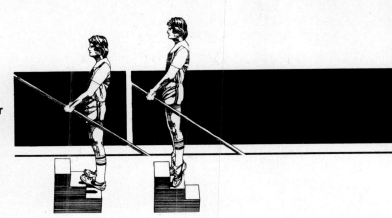

FRUIT WITH CREAMY BANANA DRESSING

½ cup small curd cream-style
    cottage cheese
1 medium banana, cut up
2 to 3 tablespoons orange juice
1 tablespoon honey
½ teaspoon sesame seed, toasted,
    or poppy seed
1 medium orange, peeled,
    sectioned, and chopped
1 medium apple, thinly sliced
1 medium banana, sliced
1 cup halved fresh strawberries
6 lettuce leaves

For dressing, in blender container combine cottage cheese, cut-up banana, orange juice, and honey. Cover and blend till smooth. Stir in sesame seed or poppy seed.

In medium bowl combine orange, apple, sliced banana, and strawberries; toss to mix. Spoon fruit onto individual lettuce-lined plates. Top each serving of fruit with 2 tablespoons dressing. Makes 6 servings.

SESAME APPLE TOSS

1 cup halved seedless
    green grapes
1 cup sliced celery
1 cup chopped apple
½ cup orange yogurt
6 bibb lettuce cups
2 teaspoons sesame seed,
    toasted

Combine grapes, celery, and apple; toss to mix. Fold in orange yogurt. Serve in lettuce cups. Sprinkle with toasted sesame seed. Makes 6 servings.

PEAR AND BLUE CHEESE SALAD

3 tablespoons sour cream with
    blue cheese
1 tablespoon plain yogurt
2 fresh medium pears
    Lemon juice
4 leaves leaf lettuce
    Paprika

Combine sour cream and yogurt; set aside. Cut each pear in half; remove core. Cut each half into 4 wedges; brush wedges with lemon juice. Arrange pear wedges on 4 lettuce-lined plates. Top each serving with 1 tablespoon yogurt mixture. Sprinkle with paprika. Makes 4 servings.

SWEET-SOUR PLUM TOSS

¼ **cup salad oil**
3 **tablespoons vinegar**
1 **tablespoon sugar**
1½ **teaspoons soy sauce**
⅛ **teaspoon ground ginger**
4 **cups torn salad greens**
4 **fresh medium plums, pitted and
   sliced**
1 **small onion, thinly sliced and
   separated into rings**
1 **cup fresh bean sprouts**

For dressing, in screw-top jar combine salad oil, vinegar, sugar, soy sauce, and ginger; cover and shake to mix. In salad bowl combine greens, plums, onion, and sprouts. Pour dressing over salad; toss to coat. Makes 6 servings.

How to grow your own sprouts

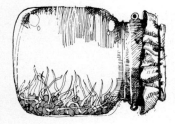

Growing your own sprouts can be fun and easy. You need only the dark corner of a kitchen shelf, two quart jars, cheesecloth, and seeds. Seeds used for sprouting that are commonly available in most grocery stores are lentils, mung beans, dried peas, pinto beans, lima beans, garbanzos (chick peas), and mustard seed. Wash and sort ½ cup of seeds, discarding damaged seeds. Soak seeds overnight in 2 cups water (seeds will swell to twice their size). Drain and rinse. Place ¼ cup of soaked seeds in each quart jar. Cover tops of jars with two layers of cheesecloth; fasten each with rubber band or string. Place jars on their sides so seeds form a shallow layer. Store in warm (68° to 75°), dark place. Rinse seeds once daily in lukewarm water. Harvest sprouts in 3 to 5 days. The whole sprout (seed, root, and stem) is edible. If you prefer to remove hulls, place sprouts in a bowl; cover with water and stir vigorously, skimming away husks as they rise to the top. Drain. Pat dry with paper toweling. Sprinkle the sprouts over tossed salads or use in cooking.

PUSH-UPS
Keep your back and legs straight and start in the "up" position. Slowly lower yourself until your chest touches the floor. Then slowly rise to the starting position. Goal: ten repetitions for women, 15 for men.

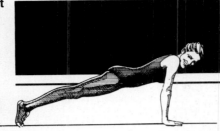

FRUIT MEDLEY SALAD

¼ **cup plain yogurt**
1 **tablespoon honey**
½ **teaspoon finely shredded lemon peel**
½ **teaspoon lemon juice**
 Dash salt
1 **cup cubed honeydew melon (¼ melon)**
1 **cup sliced fresh strawberries**
1 **medium banana, sliced**
1 **medium apple, sliced**
6 **leaves leaf lettuce**

For honey dressing combine yogurt, honey, lemon peel, lemon juice, and salt. Chill.

Combine melon, strawberries, banana, and apple. For each serving, place about ⅔ cup fruit mixture on a lettuce-lined plate. Spoon about 1 tablespoon honey dressing atop each serving. Makes 6 servings.

BANANA LOGS

3 **ounces Neufchâtel cheese, softened**
2 **tablespoons chopped raisins**
2 **teaspoons brown sugar**
⅛ **teaspoon ground cinnamon**
3 **medium bananas**
6 **leaves leaf lettuce**
2 **to 3 tablespoons orange juice**
4 **teaspoons chopped walnuts**

Divide cheese in half. Combine half of the cheese, the raisins, brown sugar, and cinnamon. Halve bananas lengthwise, then crosswise. For each serving, spread a banana quarter with about 2 teaspoons cheese mixture and top with another banana quarter; place on individual lettuce-lined plate. Combine the remaining Neufchâtel cheese and enough orange juice to make of drizzling consistency; spoon over bananas. Sprinkle with walnuts. Makes 6 servings.

CITRUS SALAD TOSS

4 **cups torn bibb lettuce**
1 **16-ounce jar refrigerated fruits for salad, drained and cut up**
½ **medium cucumber, thinly sliced**
⅓ **cup lemon yogurt**
6 **tablespoons shelled sunflower seed**

In salad bowl combine lettuce, fruits for salad, and cucumber. In small bowl combine yogurt and sunflower seed; mix well. Pour yogurt mixture over salad; toss to coat. Makes 4 servings.

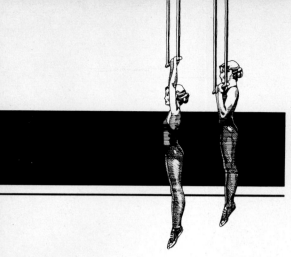

CHIN-UPS
Grasp the bar with your palms facing you. Bend your arms and pull yourself up until your chin is over the bar. Lower till your arms are straight and repeat the exercise. Chin-ups can also be done with palms facing away from you, but this may be more difficult. Goal: five repetitions for women, ten for men.

ITALIAN SCALLOP SALAD

Chill this salad at least 2 hours to allow the scallops and vegetables time to absorb the flavor of the Italian dressing—

1 **pound fresh *or* frozen scallops**
2 **cups water**
2 **tablespoons lemon juice**
½ **teaspoon salt**
1 **bay leaf**
1 **9-ounce package frozen Italian green beans, cooked and drained**
1 **cup coarsely chopped tomatoes**
½ **cup sliced celery**
½ **cup sliced fresh mushrooms**
2 **tablespoons sliced green onion**
½ **cup low-calorie Italian salad dressing**
2 **cups torn lettuce**

Thaw scallops, if frozen. In saucepan bring water, lemon juice, salt, and bay leaf to boiling; add scallops and return to boiling. Reduce heat; simmer 2 to 3 minutes. Drain and cool; slice scallops.

Combine scallops, green beans, tomato, celery, mushrooms, and onion. Pour Italian dressing over scallop mixture, tossing to coat. Cover; chill at least 2 hours, stirring occasionally. To serve, remove scallop mixture from dressing and arrange over torn lettuce. Makes 4 servings.

GARDEN TUNA SALAD

2 **6½-ounce cans tuna (water pack), drained and flaked**
1 **cup thinly sliced celery**
1 **cup coarsely shredded zucchini**
½ **cup coarsely shredded carrot**
⅓ **cup sliced radish**
⅓ **cup dairy sour cream**
⅓ **cup plain yogurt**
1 **tablespoon lemon juice**
¼ **teaspoon dried dillweed**
4 **lettuce cups**

In a bowl combine tuna, celery, zucchini, carrot, and radish; toss lightly to mix. For dressing, in separate bowl combine sour cream, yogurt, lemon juice, and dillweed. Season with salt and pepper. Chill tuna mixture and dressing. Serve tuna mixture in lettuce cups with dressing atop. Makes 4 servings.

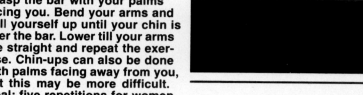

Italian Scallop Salad, Buttermilk-Blue Cheese Dressing (see recipe, page 78), Zesty Tomato Dressing, and Diet Thousand Island Dressing (see recipes, page 79) ▶

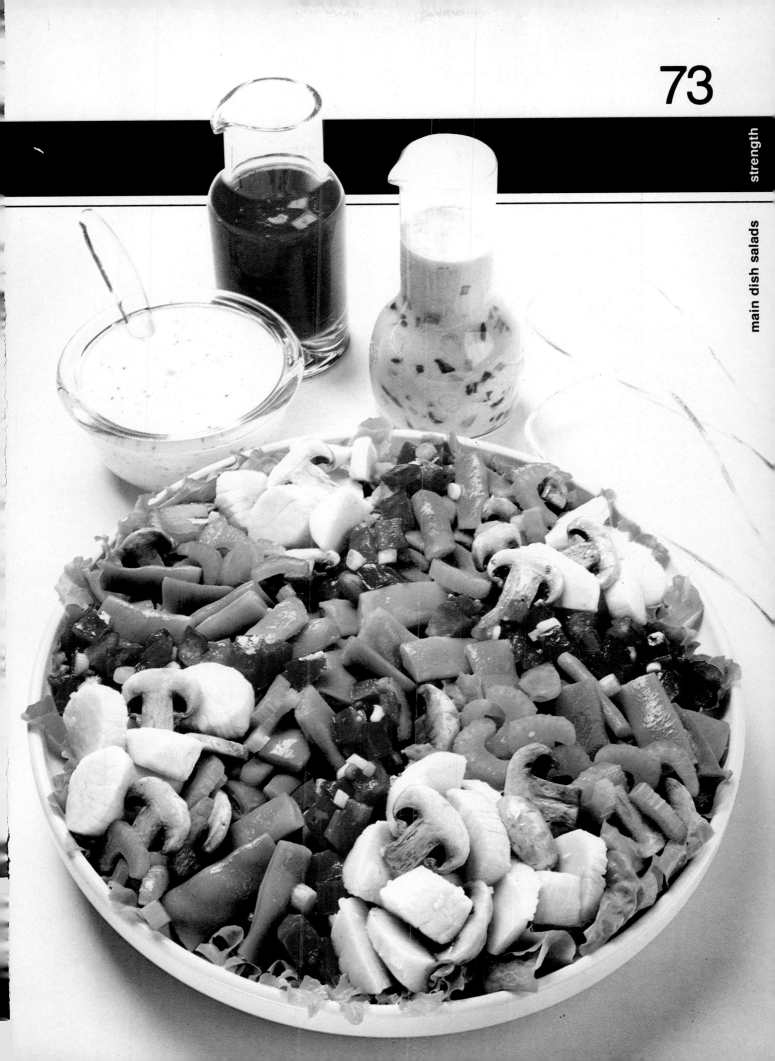

PEACH LUNCHEON SALAD

If you don't serve this salad immediately, keep the color of the peaches bright by brushing the fruit with lemon juice—

½ **cup plain yogurt**
4 **teaspoons skim milk**
1 **teaspoon white wine vinegar**
¼ **teaspoon curry powder**
2 **cups chopped cooked chicken**
¼ **cup sliced celery**
¼ **cup sliced green onion**
4 **leaves leaf lettuce**
2 **large peaches**

For dressing, in a small bowl combine yogurt and milk. Stir in vinegar, curry powder, and dash *salt*. In a bowl combine chicken, celery, and green onion; stir in enough dressing to moisten (about ⅓ cup). Chill chicken mixture and remaining dressing. To serve, line 4 individual salad plates with lettuce leaves. Peel peaches and cut each into 8 wedges. Arrange 4 peach wedges in spoke fashion on each plate. Place about ½ cup chicken mixture atop peaches in center of each salad plate. Drizzle remaining dressing over salads. Makes 4 servings.

COTTAGE TOMATO CUPS (pictured on page 30)

Serve this side-dish luncheon salad with cheddar cheese and a selection from the bread-cereal group to provide a well-balanced meal—

6 **medium tomatoes**
¾ **cup dry cottage cheese**
¼ **cup low-calorie mayonnaise**
¼ **cup chopped cucumber**
¼ **cup thinly sliced radish**
¼ **cup chopped green pepper**
2 **tablespoons sliced green onion**
½ **teaspoon dried basil, crushed**
¼ **teaspoon garlic salt**
1 **4½-ounce can shrimp, rinsed
   and drained**
6 **leaves bibb lettuce**

Place tomatoes, stem end down, on cutting surface. With sharp knife cut tomato into 6 wedges, cutting to but not through the base of the tomato. Cover and chill. In bowl combine cottage cheese and mayonnaise; mix well. Stir in cucumber, radish, green pepper, green onion, basil, and garlic salt. Gently fold in shrimp. Place the tomatoes on individual lettuce-lined salad plates and spread the wedges apart. Place about ⅓ cup cottage cheese mixture in the center of each tomato. Makes 6 servings.

Crisp, cold relishes for color and crunch

As a salad, or to accompany a meal, try relishes such as carrot curls, green pepper rings, cucumber and zucchini cut into julienne strips, cauliflower and broccoli flowerets, and radish roses. To keep the crunch in relishes, chill in ice water several hours or serve atop crushed ice.

NECK EXERCISES
Clasp hands behind head. For five seconds slowly pull head forward while resisting with neck. Then put palms on forehead and for five seconds push head back while resisting with neck. Finally, put right hand against right side of head. For ten seconds push head to left while resisting with neck. Repeat for left side. Goal: one repetition of each exercise.

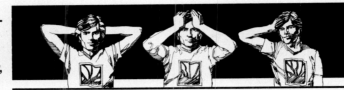

CHICKEN-ASPARAGUS TOSS

Blue cheese, chicken, and asparagus make an uncommon flavor combination—

1½ cups chopped cooked chicken
1 10-ounce package frozen asparagus spears, thawed, drained, and cut into 2-inch pieces
1 cup thinly sliced cucumber
1 cup cubed Swiss cheese (4 ounces)
1 large tomato, cut into 8 wedges
¼ cup plain yogurt
¼ cup dairy sour cream
¼ cup crumbled blue cheese (1 ounce)
¼ teaspoon garlic salt
¼ teaspoon celery seed
Dash pepper
4 lettuce cups

In large bowl combine chicken, asparagus, cucumber, cheese, and tomato. For dressing, in small bowl combine yogurt, sour cream, blue cheese, garlic salt, celery seed, and pepper; mix well. Pour dressing over chicken mixture and toss to coat. Serve in lettuce cups. Makes 4 servings.

CHICKEN-PINEAPPLE SALAD

1 small fresh pineapple *or* one 20-ounce can pineapple chunks (juice pack), drained
8 ounces cooked chicken breast meat, cut into julienne strips
1 cup halved fresh strawberries
1 cup seeded halved grapes
½ cup celery cut into ½-inch pieces
4 leaves leaf lettuce
¾ cup plain yogurt
2 teaspoons snipped fresh mint
1 teaspoon sugar

If using fresh pineapple, cut peel from pineapple; core and cut into chunks (should have about 2¼ cups pineapple chunks). In large bowl combine fresh or canned pineapple, chicken, strawberries, grapes, and celery; mix well. Place chicken mixture on 4 lettuce-lined salad plates. In small bowl combine yogurt, mint, and sugar; drizzle about 3 tablespoons yogurt mixture over each serving. Makes 4 servings.

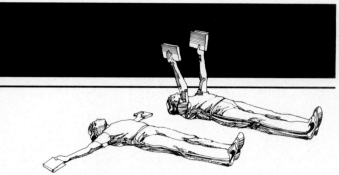

CHEST MUSCLE EXERCISE
Lie on your back atop a bench or on the floor. Hold a weight (heavy book, sand-filled container, or a light dumbbell) in each hand. Start with arms extended above you with elbows slightly bent. Slowly lower your arms to the side and then bring back up to the starting position. Goal: ten repetitions for men and women.

DILLED VEGETABLE MEDLEY SALAD

1½ cups thinly sliced cucumber
½ cup sliced radish
¼ cup sliced green onion
¼ cup plain yogurt
2 tablespoons dairy sour cream
2 tablespoons tarragon vinegar
2 teaspoons snipped fresh dill
   or ½ teaspoon dried dillweed
Dash salt
4 leaves leaf lettuce

Combine cucumber, radish, and onion. In small bowl combine yogurt, sour cream, tarragon vinegar, fresh or dried dill, and the salt; add to vegetable mixture and toss to coat. Chill thoroughly. Serve on individual lettuce-lined plates. Makes 4 servings.

GARDEN VINAIGRETTE SALAD

½ head cauliflower, broken into small flowerets (3 cups)
2 medium zucchini, sliced
1 medium green pepper, cut into strips
½ cup Vinaigrette Dressing (see recipe, page 79)
12 cherry tomatoes
   Lettuce leaves

In covered saucepan cook cauliflower flowerets in small amount of boiling, lightly salted water for 2 minutes. Add zucchini and cook 2 minutes more or till vegetables are crisp-tender. Drain. Combine cooked vegetables and green pepper. Pour Vinaigrette Dressing over vegetable mixture; toss to coat vegetables. Cover and refrigerate several hours or overnight, stirring occasionally. At serving time, halve tomatoes and add to vegetable mixture; toss gently to coat. To serve, lift vegetables from dressing with slotted spoon and place in lettuce-lined bowl. Makes 8 servings.

ZUCCHINI SALAD   (pictured on page 67)

2 small zucchini, cut into julienne strips
⅓ cup vinegar
3 tablespoons salad oil
1 tablespoon finely chopped onion
1 tablespoon chopped pimiento
1 clove garlic, minced
¼ teaspoon dried tarragon, crushed
⅛ teaspoon salt
   Dash pepper

Place zucchini in a bowl. For marinade, combine vinegar, salad oil, onion, pimiento, garlic, tarragon, salt, and pepper; mix well and pour over zucchini. Cover; refrigerate several hours or overnight, stirring occasionally. To serve, lift zucchini mixture from liquid with slotted spoon. Makes 4 servings.

MARINATED POTATO SALAD

⅓ cup low-calorie Italian salad
    dressing
2 cups hot cooked cubed potatoes
    (1 pound)
½ cup bias-sliced celery
½ cup thinly sliced red onion,
    separated into rings
¼ cup sliced radish
2 tablespoons chopped green
    pepper
½ teaspoon salt
¼ teaspoon dried dillweed
2 tablespoons snipped parsley

In a large bowl pour dressing over hot potatoes; mix gently to coat. Cover and marinate in refrigerator for at least 2 hours. Add celery, onion, radish, green pepper, salt, and dillweed; toss gently to combine. Sprinkle with parsley. Makes 6 servings.

BULGUR SALAD

1 cup boiling water
⅓ cup bulgur wheat
1 medium tomato, peeled and
    chopped
½ cup chopped cucumber
¼ cup snipped parsley
2 tablespoons sliced green onion
2 tablespoons lemon juice
4 teaspoons salad oil
¼ teaspoon salt
    Dash pepper
2½ cups shredded lettuce

Pour boiling water over bulgur wheat; let stand for 1 hour. Drain well, pressing out excess water. Combine bulgur, tomato, cucumber, parsley, onion, lemon juice, salad oil, salt, and pepper; mix well. Cover and chill several hours. For each serving, spoon about ½ cup bulgur mixture atop ½ cup shredded lettuce in individual salad bowls. Makes 5 servings.

TOMATO VEGETABLE ASPIC

1 envelope unflavored gelatin
1½ cups tomato juice
3 tablespoons vinegar
1 tablespoon sugar
½ cup shredded zucchini
½ cup finely chopped cabbage
¼ cup shredded carrot

In saucepan soften gelatin in ½ cup of the tomato juice. Cook and stir over low heat till gelatin is dissolved. Add remaining tomato juice, the vinegar, and sugar, stirring till sugar is dissolved. Stir in zucchini, cabbage, and carrot; mix well. Pour into 3-cup mold or four 6-ounce custard cups. Chill several hours or till firm. Unmold to serve. Makes 4 servings.

CAULIFLOWER SLAW

2 cups chopped cauliflower
½ cup shredded carrot
¼ cup chopped onion
½ cup plain yogurt
2 tablespoons salad dressing
2 teaspoons sugar
2 teaspoons lemon juice
¼ teaspoon celery seed
⅛ teaspoon salt
   Snipped parsley

In a large bowl combine cauliflower, carrot, and onion. In a small bowl combine yogurt, salad dressing, sugar, lemon juice, celery seed, and salt; mix well. Pour yogurt mixture over vegetables; toss to coat. Garnish with parsley. Makes 6 servings.

CONFETTI SLAW

2 cups shredded cabbage
¼ cup chopped green pepper
¼ cup chopped celery
2 tablespoons chopped pimiento
2 tablespoons vinegar
1 tablespoon sugar
1 tablespoon water
¼ teaspoon salt

Combine cabbage, green pepper, celery, and pimiento. Combine vinegar, sugar, water, and salt, stirring till sugar is dissolved. Pour vinegar mixture over vegetables; toss to coat. Cover and chill. Makes 4 servings.

BUTTERMILK-BLUE CHEESE DRESSING   (pictured on page 73)

1 cup plain yogurt
½ cup buttermilk
3 ounces blue cheese,
   crumbled (¾ cup)
1 teaspoon celery seed
¼ teaspoon salt
¼ teaspoon dried tarragon, crushed
   Dash pepper

In mixing bowl combine yogurt and buttermilk; stir in blue cheese, celery seed, salt, tarragon, and pepper. Transfer to storage container; cover and chill. Makes about 2 cups.

PULL-OVER
Lie on your back atop a bench or on the floor. Hold a weight (heavy book, sand-filled container, or a light dumbbell) in each hand. Start with arms extended above you with elbows slightly bent. Let arms go slowly back over your head to the floor, then return to starting position. Goal: ten repetitions for men and women. Good for chest muscles.

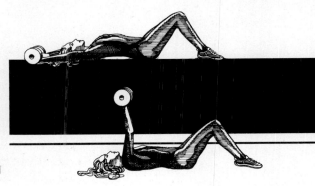

VINAIGRETTE DRESSING

⅔ cup vinegar
½ cup salad oil
2 teaspoons dry mustard
1 teaspoon paprika
1 teaspoon dried basil, crushed
1 teaspoon dried oregano, crushed
½ teaspoon dried dillweed
⅛ teaspoon bottled hot pepper sauce

In a screw-top jar combine vinegar, salad oil, dry mustard, paprika, basil, oregano, dillweed, and hot pepper sauce; cover and shake well to mix. Chill. Shake again just before serving. Chill to store. Makes about 1 cup.

DIET SALAD DRESSING   (Thousand Island variation pictured on pages 21 and 73)

1 tablespoon all-purpose flour
1 tablespoon sugar
1 teaspoon dry mustard
½ teaspoon salt
Dash ground red pepper
¾ cup skim milk
2 slightly beaten egg yolks
3 tablespoons vinegar

In saucepan combine flour, sugar, dry mustard, salt, and red pepper; stir in milk. Cook and stir till thickened and bubbly. Gradually stir hot mixture into egg yolks. Return mixture to saucepan; cook and stir 2 minutes more. Cover surface with waxed paper; cool 10 to 15 minutes. Remove waxed paper; stir in vinegar. Transfer to storage container; cover and chill. Makes ¾ cup.

Diet Thousand Island Dressing: Prepare Diet Salad Dressing as above. In small mixing bowl combine ½ cup of the *Diet Salad Dressing*, 1 tablespoon sliced *green onion*, 1 tablespoon chopped *green pepper*, 1 tablespoon chopped *pimiento*, 1 tablespoon *catsup or chili sauce*, and 1 teaspoon prepared *horseradish*; mix well. Transfer to storage container; cover and chill. Makes ⅔ cup.

ZESTY TOMATO DRESSING   (pictured on page 73)

1 8-ounce can tomato sauce
4 teaspoons vinegar
2 teaspoons Worcestershire sauce
1 teaspoon sugar
1 teaspoon grated onion
¾ teaspoon prepared horseradish

In screw-top jar combine tomato sauce, vinegar, Worcestershire sauce, sugar, onion, horseradish, ¼ teaspoon *salt*, and dash *pepper*. Cover; shake to mix. Chill to store. Makes about 1 cup.

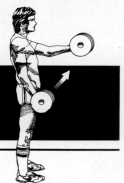

FORWARD LIFT
Stand erect with arms down at your sides. Hold a weight (a heavy book for women or a five- to ten-pound weight for men) in each hand. Raise your arms forward to the shoulder level, moving *very slowly*. Keep your arms straight. Lower your arms to the original position slowly. Goal: ten repetitions.

DESSERTS, SNACKS, & BEVERAGES

CHOCOLATE MOUSSE MERINGUES

Individual Meringue Shells
¼ cup sugar
3 tablespoons unsweetened cocoa powder
1 teaspoon unflavored gelatin
½ cup evaporated skimmed milk
2 slightly beaten egg yolks
Dash salt
½ teaspoon vanilla
1 1½-ounce envelope dessert topping mix
½ cup skim milk
5 fresh strawberries, halved

Prepare Individual Meringue Shells. Cool thoroughly.

In a heavy saucepan combine sugar, cocoa powder, and gelatin. Stir in evaporated skimmed milk, egg yolks, and salt, mixing till well blended. Cook and stir over low heat about 3 minutes or till slightly thickened; stir in vanilla. Cool for 5 to 10 minutes. (If mixture appears curdled, stir well with wire whisk.)

In small mixer bowl combine dessert topping mix and skim milk; beat with electric mixer till soft peaks form. Fold *half* of the dessert topping into the chocolate mixture; cover and chill. Cover and chill remaining topping till serving time. At serving time, spoon *1 tablespoon* of the whipped dessert topping, then *3 tablespoons* of the chocolate mixture into each meringue shell. Top each with a strawberry half. Makes 10 servings.

Individual Meringue Shells: Let 2 *egg whites* come to room temperature. For meringue, in small mixer bowl combine the egg whites, ½ teaspoon *cream of tartar*, ½ teaspoon *vanilla*, and dash *salt*. Beat on high speed of electric mixer till soft peaks form. Gradually add ½ cup *sugar*, beating till stiff peaks form. Line a baking sheet with plain brown paper. Draw ten 2½-inch circles on paper; place a mound of meringue on each. Using back of spoon, shape meringue into shells. Bake in 300° oven for 35 mintues. (For crisper meringues, turn off oven. Dry meringue shells in oven with door closed about 1 hour more.)

HONEYDEW ICE

1 teaspoon unflavored gelatin
2 tablespoons water
4 cups cubed honeydew melon (1 medium)
2 tablespoons lime juice
2 tablespoons honey

In 1-cup glass measure or a custard cup soften gelatin in water; place in pan of water. Heat and stir till gelatin is dissolved. In blender container combine *1 cup* of the melon cubes, the lime juice, honey, and the gelatin mixture. Cover and blend at high speed for 30 seconds or till smooth. Add remaining melon; cover and blend at high speed 30 to 45 seconds or till smooth. Pour into an 8x8x2-inch pan. Freeze till almost firm. In chilled large mixer bowl beat mixture at high speed of electric mixer till smooth. Return to pan; freeze several hours or till firm. To serve, let stand 15 to 20 minutes at room temperature. Scrape surface and spoon into serving dishes. If desired, garnish with lime twists. Serves 6.

Chocolate Mousse Meringues, Honeydew Ice ▶

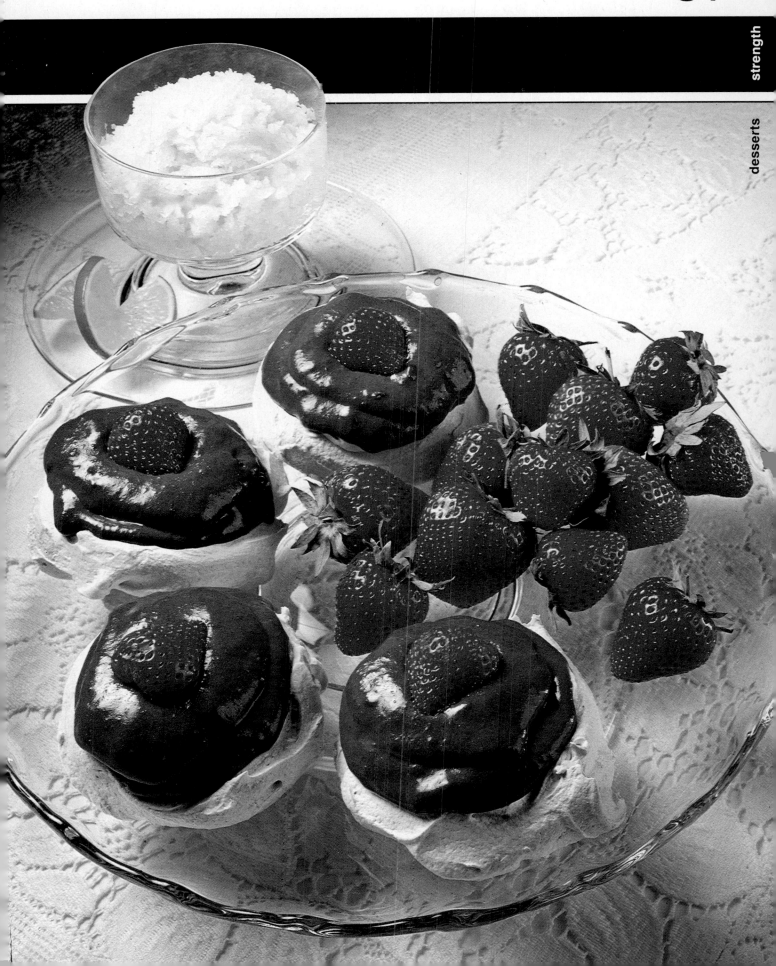

ORANGE YOGURT PIE   (pictured on page 30)

1⅓ cups flaked coconut (1 3½-
    ounce can)
1 tablespoon butter *or* margarine,
    melted
1 20-ounce can crushed pineapple
    (juice pack)
1 envelope unflavored gelatin
2 8-ounce cartons orange yogurt

Place 1¼ *cups* of the coconut in a bowl; toss with melted butter or margarine. Press on the bottom and up sides of a 9-inch pie plate. Bake in a 325° oven about 15 minutes or till golden. Cool on wire rack. Place remaining coconut in a shallow pan and toast in 325° oven about 1 minute. Set aside.

Drain pineapple, reserving juice. Set fruit aside. Add water, if necessary, to reserved juice to make ¾ cup liquid. In small saucepan soften gelatin in the pineapple liquid. Cook and stir over low heat till gelatin is dissolved. Chill till partially set (consistency of unbeaten egg whites). Beat partially set gelatin mixture till fluffy. Fold in yogurt and drained pineapple. Pile into cooled crust. Garnish with reserved toasted coconut. Chill till firm. Serves 8.

ORANGE SPONGE CAKE   (pictured on the cover)

1 cup sifted cake flour
1¼ cups sifted powdered sugar
5 egg yolks
¼ teaspoon salt
1 tablespoon finely shredded
    orange peel
5 egg whites
1 teaspoon vanilla
½ teaspoon cream of tartar
1 cup orange juice
1 tablespoon honey
¾ teaspoon almond extract

Combine cake flour and ½ *cup* of the sifted powdered sugar; set aside. In small mixer bowl beat egg yolks on high speed of electric mixer about 6 minutes or till thick and lemon-colored. Gradually add the remaining ¾ cup sifted powdered sugar and the salt, beating constantly about 4 minutes. Stir in the shredded orange peel.

Wash beaters. In large mixer bowl beat egg whites, vanilla, and cream of tartar till soft peaks form. Gently fold yolk mixture into whites. Sift flour mixture over egg mixture, ⅓ at a time, and fold in gently. Turn into an *ungreased* 9-inch tube pan. Bake in 325° oven about 55 minutes or till cake springs back and leaves no imprint when lightly touched. Invert cake in pan; cool thoroughly. Remove from pan.

With a long-tined fork, poke holes in top of cake at 1-inch intervals. For syrup, in a saucepan combine orange juice and honey. Simmer for 5 minutes. Remove from heat; stir in almond extract. Spoon syrup liquid evenly over cake, a small amount at a time, allowing cake to absorb the syrup. Chill, if desired. Makes 16 servings.

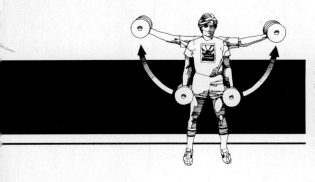

GINGERBREAD WITH LEMON SAUCE

1 cup all-purpose flour
1 teaspoon baking soda
¼ teaspoon ground ginger
¼ teaspoon ground cinnamon
¼ teaspoon ground nutmeg
¼ cup packed brown sugar
¼ cup water
¼ cup light molasses
½ teaspoon finely shredded lemon peel (set aside)
2 tablespoons lemon juice
Non-stick vegetable spray coating
¼ cup sugar
1 tablespoon cornstarch
⅛ teaspoon salt
⅛ teaspoon ground nutmeg
¾ cup water
2 tablespoons lemon juice

In medium mixing bowl stir together the flour, baking soda, ginger, cinnamon, and ¼ teaspoon nutmeg. Mix well. In small bowl combine brown sugar, the ¼ cup water, molasses, and 2 tablespoons lemon juice; stir into flour mixture just till blended. Quickly pour batter into 3 soup cans (2½-inch diameter) sprayed with non-stick vegetable spray coating. Cover with foil. Bake in 350° oven for 20 to 25 minutes or till wooden pick inserted in center comes out clean. Cool 10 minutes; remove from cans.

Meanwhile, for lemon sauce, in small saucepan combine sugar, cornstarch, salt, the ⅛ teaspoon nutmeg, and lemon peel. Stir in the ¾ cup water. Cook and stir till thickened and bubbly. Stir in 2 tablespoons lemon juice. Serve gingerbread topped with lemon sauce. Makes 9 servings.

APPLE SOUFFLÉ

Non-stick vegetable spray coating
2 egg yolks
4 teaspoons butter *or* margarine
2 tablespoons all-purpose flour
¼ cup skim milk
2 tablespoons frozen apple juice concentrate, thawed
1 tablespoon apple brandy *or* brandy
2 egg whites
2 tablespoons sugar

Spray the bottom and sides of a 1-quart soufflé dish and a foil collar with the non-stick vegetable spray coating. Attach the foil collar around the top of the soufflé dish. In a small mixer bowl beat the egg yolks on high speed of electric mixer about 6 minutes or till thick and lemon-colored; set aside. In saucepan melt butter or margarine; stir in flour. Add the milk all at once. Cook and stir till mixture is very thick and bubbly. Remove from heat. Stir in apple juice concentrate and brandy. Slowly add egg yolks, stirring constantly. Wash beaters. In large mixer bowl beat egg whites till soft peaks form. Gradually add sugar, beating till stiff peaks form; gently fold into yolk mixture. Turn into soufflé dish. Bake in 300° oven about 60 minutes. Serve immediately. Serves 4.

PEACH TORTE

Non-stick vegetable spray
  coating
⅔ cup sifted cake flour
¾ cup sifted powdered sugar
3 egg yolks
¼ teaspoon salt
3 egg whites
½ teaspoon vanilla
¼ teaspoon cream of tartar
¼ teaspoon almond extract
1 16-ounce can peach slices
  (juice pack)
2 tablespoons sugar
1 tablespoon cornstarch
⅛ teaspoon almond extract
1 1½-ounce envelope dessert
  topping mix
½ cup skim milk

Spray two 8x1½-inch round baking pans with non-stick vegetable spray coating; line with waxed paper. Set aside. In a bowl combine flour and ¼ *cup* of the powdered sugar; set aside. Beat egg yolks on high speed of electric mixer about 6 minutes or till thick and lemon-colored. Gradually add ¼ *cup* of the powdered sugar and the salt, beating constantly. Wash beaters thoroughly. Beat egg whites, vanilla, cream of tartar, and ¼ teaspoon almond extract till soft peaks form. Gradually add the remaining ¼ cup powdered sugar, beating till stiff peaks form. Gently fold yolk mixture into whites. Sift flour mixture over egg mixture, ⅓ at a time, folding in gently just till blended. Turn into the prepared pans. Bake in a 325° oven about 20 minutes or till cakes spring back and leave no imprint when lightly touched. (Cakes will be light in color.) Invert cakes in pans; cool completely. Remove cakes from pans; remove waxed paper.

Meanwhile, drain peaches, reserving ½ cup juice. Coarsely chop peach slices; set aside. In saucepan combine sugar and cornstarch. Stir in the reserved peach juice. Cook and stir till thickened and bubbly; cook and stir 1 to 2 minutes more. Remove from heat. Stir in peaches and ⅛ teaspoon almond extract. Cover and cool.

Combine dessert topping mix and milk; beat with electric mixer till soft peaks form. To assemble torte, place one cake layer on serving plate; spoon *half* of the peach mixture over cake. Top with *half* of the dessert topping. Add second cake layer. Pipe or spread remaining dessert topping in a spiral atop cake. Fill spiral with remaining peach mixture. Chill. Makes 10 servings.

BERRY-MELON FRUIT CUP (pictured on page 21)

2 cups sliced fresh strawberries
2 cups cantaloupe balls
  (1 medium)
2 tablespoons shredded coconut,
  toasted
⅓ cup orange juice
1 tablespoon honey
1 tablespoon orange liqueur
¼ teaspoon ground ginger

In large bowl combine strawberries, cantaloupe, and coconut; toss to mix. In small bowl combine orange juice, honey, orange liqueur, and ginger; add to fruit mixture, stirring to coat. Cover and chill about 1 hour. Makes 8 servings.

BACK LIFT
Lie on your stomach with hands
clasped behind your neck. Have a
partner hold your ankles. Raise
your trunk and head as far as
possible. Try to work up to raising your chin 18 to 24 inches
from the floor. Hold the position
five seconds. Goal: three to five
repetitions. Start gradually;
progress is slow.

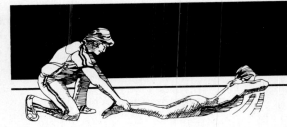

MANDARIN RICE PUDDING

  2 **cups skim milk**
  ⅓ **cup long grain rice**
  1 **beaten egg yolk**
  ¼ **teaspoon finely shredded**
      orange peel (set aside)
  2 **tablespoons orange juice**
  2 **tablespoons sugar**
  ¼ **teaspoon salt**
  1 **teaspoon vanilla**
  3 **egg whites**
  ¼ **teaspoon cream of tartar**
  2 **tablespoons sugar**
  1 **11-ounce can mandarin orange**
      sections, chilled and drained
     Mint sprigs

In medium saucepan combine milk and rice. Bring to boiling.
Reduce heat; cook, covered, over low heat for 20 minutes, stirring
occasionally. Uncover; cook 5 minutes more.

In a small bowl combine egg yolk and orange juice; stir in 2
tablespoons sugar and the salt. Gradually stir about *1 cup* of the
hot rice mixture into yolk mixture; return all to saucepan. Bring
mixture to a gentle boil. Cook and stir over low heat about 2
minutes or till slightly thickened. Remove from heat; stir in vanilla
and orange peel. Cool thoroughly.

In a small mixer bowl beat egg whites and cream of tartar on
high speed of electric mixer till soft peaks form. Gradually add 2
tablespoons sugar, beating till stiff peaks form. Fold egg whites
into cooled rice mixture. Set aside 6 orange sections for garnish.
Fold remaining orange sections into rice mixture. Cover and chill
for several hours. To serve, garnish with reserved orange sections
and mint sprigs. Makes 6 servings.

ORANGE CHIFFON DESSERT

  3 **tablespoons sugar**
  1 **envelope unflavored**
      gelatin
     Dash salt
  1 **cup orange juice**
  ¼ **cup water**
  3 **beaten egg yolks**
  1 **11-ounce can mandarin**
      orange sections
  3 **egg whites**
  ½ **of a 4-ounce container frozen**
      whipped dessert topping,
      thawed

In saucepan combine sugar, unflavored gelatin, and salt; stir in
orange juice and water. Stir in beaten egg yolks. Cook and stir
over medium heat 10 to 12 minutes or till slightly thickened and
bubbly. Remove from heat. Chill, stirring occasionally, just till mixture mounds slightly when spooned.

Drain mandarin orange sections; reserve 8 orange sections for
garnish. Chop remaining orange sections; fold into gelatin mixture. Beat egg whites till stiff peaks form; fold into gelatin mixture.
Turn mixture into eight 6-ounce custard cups. Cover and chill till
firm. If desired, invert onto plate. Top each with about 1 tablespoon
whipped dessert topping and a reserved mandarin orange section. Makes 8 servings.

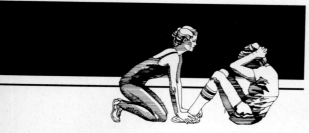

SIT-UPS
Have someone hold your feet or put them under a heavy couch or chair. Bend your knees. Clasp your hands behind your neck, elbows pointed ahead (pointing elbows straight out is more difficult). If you find either of those positions too difficult, keep your arms at your side. Tuck your chin onto your chest and roll up and back at a moderate pace.
Goal: 15 sit-ups.

FROZEN ORANGE MIST

¼ teaspoon finely shredded
    orange peel
1 cup orange juice
¼ cup sugar
1 tablespoon lemon juice
1 cup *reconstituted* nonfat dry milk
⅔ cup evaporated skimmed milk

Combine orange peel, orange juice, sugar, and lemon juice; stir till sugar dissolves. Gradually add to *reconstituted* nonfat dry milk, stirring constantly. Pour into 10x6x2- or 8x8x2-inch dish; freeze till firm. Meanwhile, pour evaporated milk into a small mixer bowl; freeze till ice crystals form around edges. Break frozen orange juice mixture into chunks; place in chilled large bowl. Beat with electric mixer till smooth.

Beat the icy cold evaporated milk with electric mixer till stiff peaks form; fold into orange juice mixture. Turn into 10x6x2- or 8x8x2-inch dish; freeze till firm. Scoop to serve. Makes 8 servings.

WAIST-WATCHERS ZABAGLIONE

3 medium pears, sliced
3 medium apples, sliced
1 tablespoon lemon juice
3 egg yolks
¼ cup cream sherry
2 tablespoons sugar
    Dash salt
½ of a 4-ounce container of frozen
    whipped dessert topping,
    thawed

Sprinkle pears and apples with lemon juice; toss to coat. Set aside. In top of double boiler beat egg yolks and sherry till combined; stir in sugar and salt. Place over boiling water (water should not touch upper pan). Beat at high speed of electric mixer for 6 to 8 minutes or till mixture thickens and mounds. When thick, place pan over ice water (if using a glass pan, transfer contents to metal bowl). Continue beating 2 to 3 minutes or till cool. Fold in whipped dessert topping. Serve over fruit immediately. Serves 8.

TOASTY OAT CRACKERS   (pictured on page 89)

1½ cups quick-cooking rolled oats
    or regular rolled oats
⅔ cup all-purpose flour
⅓ cup wheat germ
1 tablespoon sugar
1 tablespoon sesame seed
½ teaspoon salt, seasoned salt,
    or garlic salt
¼ cup butter *or* margarine
½ cup water

Place quick-cooking rolled oats or regular rolled oats in a blender container or food processor bowl. Cover and blend about 1 minute or till oats are evenly ground.

In a mixing bowl combine oats, flour, wheat germ, sugar, sesame seed, and salt. Cut in butter till mixture resembles coarse crumbs. Gradually add water, mixing till dry ingredients are moistened. Shape dough into a 9-inch-long roll. Wrap and chill for several hours. Cut into ⅛-inch slices; place on ungreased baking sheet. Flatten till very thin with tines of a fork. Bake in 375° oven about 12 minutes or till edges are brown. Remove and cool on wire rack. Makes about 72.

CREAMY CHEESE SNACKS

4 ounces Neufchâtel cheese,
   softened
1 tablespoon sliced green onion
¼ teaspoon celery seed
   Dash garlic powder
24 melba toast rounds
   Paprika

In small mixer bowl combine cheese, green onion, celery seed and garlic powder. Beat with electric mixer till smooth. Spread about *1 teaspoon* of the cheese mixture on each toast round; place on ungreased baking sheet. Sprinkle with paprika. Broil 5 inches from heat about 1 minute or just till cheese is hot. Serve immediately. Makes 24.

BRAN-APPLE SQUARES

   Non-stick vegetable spray
      coating
1 cup 40% bran flakes
½ cup wheat germ
½ cup nonfat dry milk powder
½ teaspoon baking powder
2 beaten eggs
½ cup packed brown sugar
½ cup peeled and finely shredded
   apple
2 tablespoons cooking oil
1 tablespoon light molasses
2 teaspoons vanilla
½ cup chopped walnuts

Spray a 9x9x2-inch baking pan with non-stick vegetable spray coating. In a large mixing bowl stir together bran flakes, wheat germ, dry milk powder, and baking powder. In a small bowl combine eggs, brown sugar, apple, oil, molasses, and vanilla. Add egg mixture to dry ingredients, mixing well. Stir in walnuts. Turn into prepared pan. Bake in 350° oven about 25 minutes. Cool on wire rack. Cut into squares. Makes 20 servings.

GARDEN VEGETABLE DIP

1 8-ounce carton plain yogurt
2 tablespoons finely chopped
   cucumber
2 tablespoons finely chopped
   green onion
1 tablespoon snipped parsley
1 tablespoon chili sauce
⅛ teaspoon garlic powder
   Dash bottled hot pepper sauce
2 cups fresh vegetable dippers*

In a bowl combine yogurt, cucumber, green onion, parsley, chili sauce, garlic powder, and hot pepper sauce; stir gently to blend. Serve with fresh vegetable dippers. Makes 4 servings.
Note: For fresh vegetable dippers use desired assortment of broccoli, carrots, cauliflower, celery, cucumber, mushrooms, cherry tomatoes, green onion, green pepper, and zucchini.

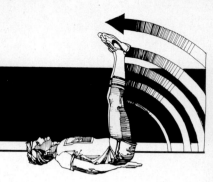

LEG RAISES
While lying on your back with hands under buttocks, palms down, slowly raise both legs together until they're perpendicular to the floor. Then slowly lower them to the floor again. You can vary the routine by slowly raising and lowering just one leg at a time, scissors fashion. Goal: 15 repetitions for each leg. Good for conditioning abdominal muscles.

PINEAPPLE YOGURT NUT LOAF

2½ cups whole wheat flour
½ cup 40% bran flakes
2 tablespoons wheat germ
1 teaspoon baking soda
1 teaspoon baking powder
  Dash salt
1 beaten egg
2 8-ounce cartons pineapple yogurt
¼ cup milk
2 tablespoons cooking oil
2 tablespoons light molasses
2 tablespoons honey
1 teaspoon lemon juice
1 cup raisins
½ cup chopped walnuts
½ cup snipped, pitted whole dates
  Non-stick vegetable spray coating

In a bowl stir together whole wheat flour, bran flakes, wheat germ, baking soda, baking powder, and salt. In a second bowl combine egg, yogurt, milk, cooking oil, molasses, honey, and lemon juice; stir into dry ingredients just till moistened. Stir in raisins, walnuts, and dates. Turn into two 7½x3½x2-inch loaf pans sprayed with non-stick vegetable spray coating. Bake in a 325° oven 50 to 60 minutes or till wooden pick inserted near center comes out clean. Cool 10 minutes on wire rack; remove from pans. Cool loaves completely on wire rack. Wrap and store overnight before slicing. Makes 2 loaves.

GAZPACHO REFRESHER

1½ cups tomato juice, chilled
3 ice cubes
¼ medium green pepper
¼ medium carrot
¼ medium cucumber
2 sprigs parsley
2 teaspoons lemon juice
  Dash garlic salt
  Few drops bottled hot pepper sauce
½ medium cucumber, cut into spears

Place tomato juice in blender container. While blending at high speed, add ice cubes, one at a time, blending till smooth. Add green pepper, carrot, the ¼ medium cucumber, parsley, lemon juice, garlic salt, and hot pepper sauce. Cover and blend at high speed about 30 seconds. Serve with cucumber spears as stirrers. Makes 4 servings.

Toasty Oat Crackers (see recipe, page 86), Pineapple Yogurt Nut Loaf, Gazpacho Refresher, Fizzy Fruit Slush (see recipe, page 90) ▶

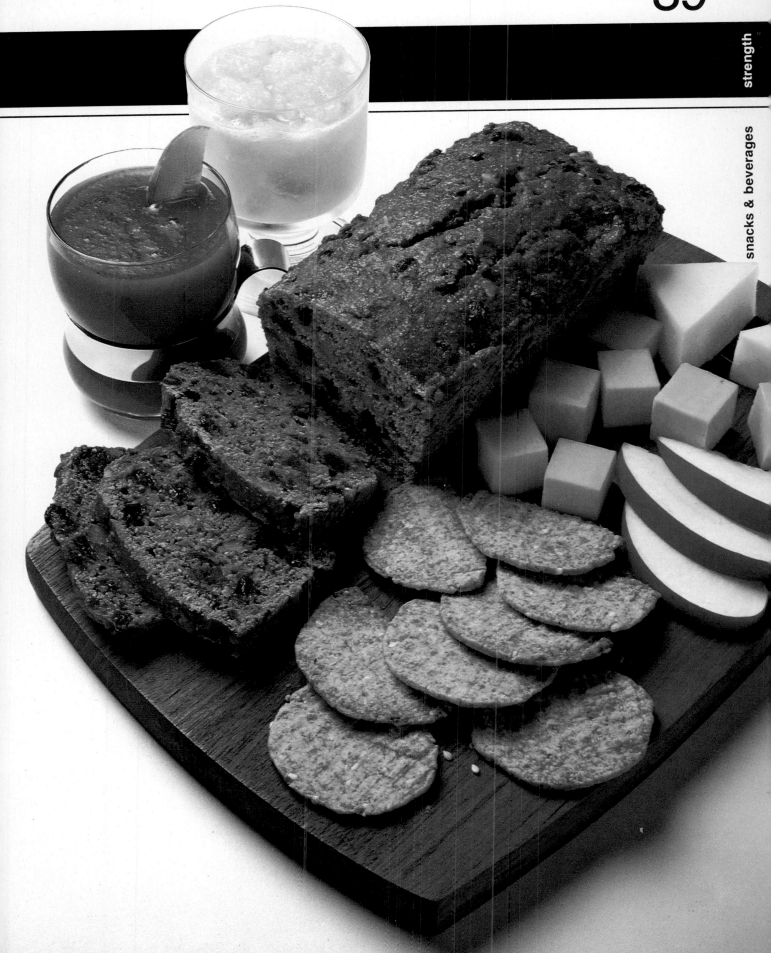

CRANBERRY WINE COOLER (pictured on page 31)

1 32-ounce bottle low-calorie
   cranberry juice cocktail,
   chilled
1 12-ounce can low-calorie
   lemon-lime carbonated
   beverage, chilled
½ cup dry red wine, chilled
   Ice cubes
8 whole fresh strawberries

In a 2-quart pitcher stir together chilled cranberry juice cocktail, carbonated beverage, and wine. Pour into ice-filled glasses. Garnish each serving with a strawberry. Makes 8 servings.

RHUBARB-APPLE CRUSH

1 pound fresh rhubarb,
   cut into ½-inch pieces (3 cups)
3 cups water
2 tablespoons honey
1 6-ounce can frozen apple juice
   concentrate
1 teaspoon grenadine syrup
   Crushed ice
1 16-ounce bottle low-calorie
   lemon-lime carbonated
   beverage, chilled

In saucepan combine rhubarb, water, and honey. Bring to boiling; reduce heat. Cover and simmer about 10 minutes or till rhubarb is very tender. Strain to remove pulp; chill the syrup and discard pulp. Combine rhubarb syrup, apple juice concentrate, and grenadine syrup; pour ½ *cup* mixture over crushed ice in each glass. Carefully pour ¼ *cup* carbonated beverage into each glass; stir. Makes 8 servings.

FIZZY FRUIT SLUSH (pictured on page 89)

1½ cups unsweetened pineapple
   juice
1½ cups water
½ of a 6-ounce can (⅓ cup) frozen
   orange juice concentrate,
   thawed
1 medium banana, pureed
1 tablespoon honey
2 12-ounce cans low-calorie lemon-
   lime carbonated beverage,
   chilled

In a 2-quart pitcher combine pineapple juice, water, orange juice concentrate, banana, and honey; mix well. Pour into 9x5-inch loaf pan. Cover and freeze several hours or till firm. To serve, thaw juice mixture at room temperature about 30 minutes or till able to scrape surface of mixture to form a slush. For each serving place ⅓ *cup* of the slush in glass and add ¼ *cup* of the carbonated beverage. Makes 12 servings.

NUTRITIONAL ANALYSIS

Recipes in this book have been nutritionally analyzed using a computer-based method. The primary source was the *Agriculture Handbook, No. 456*, published by the U.S. Dept. of Agriculture.

Use the information in this chart to plan menus to meet your daily nutritional and caloric needs. In making the analysis, suggested garnishes were not included. Also, for recipes containing two

or more ingredient options, only the first ingredient listed was used in obtaining the nutritional data. Values for cooked lean meat, trimmed of fat, were used in analyzing main dish meat recipes.

	Per Serving						Percent U.S. RDA Per Serving							
	Calories	Protein gms.	Carbohydrate gms.	Fat gms.	Sodium mgs.	Potassium mgs.	Protein	Vitamin A	Vitamin C	Thiamin	Riboflavin	Niacin	Calcium	Iron
Beverages														
Cranberry Wine Cooler (p. 90)	43	0	23	0	2	57	0	0	52	1	2	1	1	4
Fizzy Fruit Slush (p. 90)	46	0	11	0	1	147	1	2	31	3	1	1	1	1
Gazpacho Refresher (p. 88)	22	1	5	0	186	255	2	26	40	4	2	4	1	6
Rhubarb-Apple Crush (p. 90)	70	1	17	0	2	313	2	5	82	7	3	3	6	3
Desserts														
Apple Soufflé (p. 83)	138	4	14	6	83	119	7	10	24	5	8	2	4	3
Berry-Melon Fruit Cup (p. 84)	52	1	11	1	6	219	1	28	86	3	3	3	2	4
Chocolate Mousse Meringues (p. 80)	126	3	21	4	37	106	5	4	8	1	7	1	6	3
Frozen Orange Mist (p. 86)	85	3	14	2	51	214	5	3	28	4	10	1	12	1
Gingerbread with Lemon Sauce (p. 83)	127	2	30	0	4	129	3	0	5	7	4	2	6	6
Honeydew Ice (p. 80)	61	1	15	0	14	293	2	1	46	3	2	4	2	3
Mandarin Rice Pudding (p. 85)	133	6	25	1	69	206	9	5	23	7	13	2	12	3
Orange Chiffon Dessert (p. 85)	88	4	12	3	23	117	6	8	38	4	4	1	2	3
Orange Sponge Cake (p. 82)	87	3	15	2	52	58	4	4	14	2	3	1	1	2
Orange Yogurt Pie (p. 82)	149	4	20	7	55	221	6	2	10	6	7	1	10	3
Peach Torte (p. 84)	131	3	22	3	30	106	5	8	2	2	5	2	3	3
Waist-Watchers Zabaglione (p. 86)	132	2	22	4	5	149	3	6	8	3	4	1	2	4
Main Dishes														
Beef and Sprout Sandwiches (p. 50)	208	21	18	6	203	461	32	15	30	11	15	21	6	19
Beef-Broccoli Stir-Fry (p. 32)	293	21	12	18	88	703	32	119	127	12	21	25	11	23
Cassoulet Soup (p. 39)	299	20	36	8	316	859	31	41	8	31	13	15	10	29
Chicken Divan (p. 45)	169	24	10	3	217	514	36	51	111	7	15	36	14	8
Chicken Marengo (p. 46)	202	25	9	6	198	473	38	9	30	6	15	48	3	13
Chicken 'n' Swiss Stacks (p. 48)	234	19	7	15	287	402	29	18	44	6	14	19	31	8
Fish and Vegetable Bake (p. 41)	201	19	16	7	263	870	30	52	79	12	7	16	10	10
Ham and Vegetable Roll-Ups (p. 48)	203	17	4	14	863	256	25	12	14	15	12	8	23	11
Hungarian Round Steak (p. 34)	259	19	15	13	167	725	30	81	19	10	16	22	8	18
Lamb-Stuffed Squash (p. 40)	364	30	42	9	551	1142	46	59	59	21	32	34	16	26
Lemon Broiled Chicken (p. 47)	164	19	1	9	70	29	29	4	9	4	9	36	1	6
Orange-Spiced Pork Chops (p. 38)	208	18	14	9	132	383	28	4	80	48	13	21	3	14
Pared Down Pizza (p. 33)	242	17	24	9	320	424	26	19	82	17	18	20	16	15

	Calories	Protein gms.	Carbohydrate gms.	Fat gms.	Sodium mgs.	Potassium mgs.	Protein	Vitamin A	Vitamin C	Thiamin	Riboflavin	Niacin	Calcium	Iron
Pastitsio (p. 40)	217	18	23	5	722	280	28	12	7	9	22	9	14	11
Pepper Beef Stew (p. 34)	243	25	24	6	641	612	38	25	123	15	18	24	4	24
Pork and Kraut Skillet (p. 37)	328	16	21	19	362	488	25	3	29	42	13	22	3	15
Pork and Vegetable Stir-Fry (p. 37)	352	26	26	16	1260	641	39	99	74	64	20	31	6	27
Pork Paprikash (p. 38)	263	20	25	9	155	320	30	7	14	45	18	22	7	16
Roast Beef Carbonnade (p. 32)	294	25	13	14	223	733	39	131	63	12	17	32	5	24
Saucy Pepper Burgers (p. 33)	221	20	12	9	522	477	30	12	92	11	14	26	4	19
Savory Sauced Chicken (p. 45)	163	21	7	6	178	195	32	16	19	6	11	38	6	9
Sesame-Skewered Scallops (p. 44)	177	19	12	6	385	625	29	15	81	11	6	9	11	16
Shrimp Jambalaya (p. 44)	284	22	21	12	356	434	34	17	37	18	7	24	6	17
Sole Florentine (p. 42)	163	21	12	4	394	792	32	115	57	11	18	13	24	15
Sweet and Sour Lamb (p. 39)	342	25	37	10	662	500	38	13	61	21	16	31	4	17
Tuna-Cauliflower Casserole (p. 41)	144	19	13	2	223	515	29	4	91	9	17	37	15	9
Tuna Tacos (p. 50)	312	24	32	10	274	376	37	17	22	10	11	46	24	20
Tuna-Zucchini Bake (p. 42)	160	18	9	6	472	350	27	10	37	5	17	23	18	7
Turkey-Broccoli Pilaf (p. 46)	267	27	23	7	346	528	42	39	85	12	16	36	7	13
Veal Sauté with Mushrooms (p. 36)	291	21	24	12	296	428	32	5	11	18	21	39	3	20
Veal Stew (p. 36)	323	30	19	13	477	878	46	60	32	18	32	57	4	28
Salads & Salad Dressings														
Apple-Banana Frost (p. 68)	66	1	15	1	15	173	2	3	23	3	4	1	4	2
Banana Logs (p. 71)	118	3	19	5	60	317	4	7	17	4	5	3	2	4
Bulgur Salad (p. 77)	87	2	12	4	112	189	3	13	28	5	3	4	2	6
Buttermilk-Blue Cheese Dressing (p. 78)	17	1	1	1	47	19	2	1	0	0	2	0	2	0
Cauliflower Slaw (p. 78)	54	2	7	3	95	189	3	22	56	4	5	2	4	3
Chicken-Asparagus Toss (p. 75)	291	30	8	16	430	636	47	32	53	13	24	37	36	15
Chicken-Pineapple Salad (p. 75)	225	25	24	4	105	713	38	8	70	11	13	44	10	12
Citrus Salad Toss (p. 71)	88	3	16	2	35	368	5	14	17	7	10	5	9	5
Confetti Slaw (p. 78)	28	1	7	0	154	155	1	3	63	3	2	1	2	3
Cottage Tomato Cups (p. 74)	116	10	9	5	224	423	16	27	67	7	8	7	7	10
Cranberry Orange Mold (p. 66)	103	2	25	0	3	109	2	2	62	4	2	1	2	3
Creamy Strawberry Mold (p. 66)	81	2	13	3	8	100	3	3	49	1	3	2	3	3
Diet Salad Dressing (p. 79)	22	1	2	1	98	29	2	2	0	1	3	0	2	1
Diet Thousand Island Dressing (p. 79)	24	1	2	1	77	39	2	3	5	1	2	0	2	1
Dilled Vegetable Medley Salad (p. 76)	33	1	4	2	17	195	2	9	19	2	4	1	5	5
Fruit Medley Salad (p. 71)	79	2	19	1	15	358	2	5	60	4	5	4	3	6
Fruit with Creamy Banana Dressing (p. 69)	94	3	19	1	43	284	5	6	49	4	6	3	3	5
Garden Tuna Salad (p. 72)	188	28	7	5	105	601	43	42	26	7	12	64	9	12
Garden Vinaigrette Salad (p. 76)	95	3	7	7	10	376	4	12	119	8	7	6	3	6
Italian Scallop Salad (p. 72)	183	29	14	3	838	949	44	26	42	15	12	14	19	28
Marinated Potato Salad (p. 77)	47	1	9	1	294	218	2	3	29	4	2	4	1	3
Peach Luncheon Salad (p. 74)	164	24	10	3	74	554	37	25	17	5	10	45	6	9
Pear and Blue Cheese Salad (p. 69)	74	1	14	2	9	167	2	5	10	2	4	1	3	3
Rainbow Fruit Salad (p. 68)	125	3	25	2	35	494	5	43	122	9	9	5	8	5
Sesame Apple Toss (p. 69)	59	2	12	1	40	255	3	8	10	3	4	2	5	5
Sparkling Cherry Berry Mold (p. 68)	35	2	7	0	2	64	3	1	24	1	1	1	1	1

Per Serving — **Percent U.S. RDA Per Serving**

	Calories	Protein gms.	Carbohydrate gms.	Fat gms.	Sodium mgs.	Potassium mgs.	Protein	Vitamin A	Vitamin C	Thiamin	Riboflavin	Niacin	Calcium	Iron
Spiced Fruit Mold (p. 66)	62	2	14	0	2	178	2	3	47	4	2	1	2	3
Sweet-Sour Plum Toss (p. 70)	129	2	12	9	117	221	2	5	17	4	4	3	2	5
Tomato Vegetable Aspic (p. 77)	44	3	9	0	190	301	4	31	39	4	3	5	2	6
Vinaigrette Dressing (p. 79)	62	0	1	7	0	10	0	0	0	0	0	0	0	0
Zesty Tomato Dressing (p. 79)	6	0	1	0	137	2	0	3	1	1	0	1	0	0
Zucchini Salad (p. 76)	105	1	4	10	7	150	1	5	24	2	3	3	2	2

Snacks

	Calories	Protein gms.	Carbohydrate gms.	Fat gms.	Sodium mgs.	Potassium mgs.	Protein	Vitamin A	Vitamin C	Thiamin	Riboflavin	Niacin	Calcium	Iron
Bran-Apple Squares (p. 87)	85	3	10	4	36	111	4	3	2	6	6	3	3	8
Creamy Cheese Snacks (p. 87)	28	1	2	2	55	10	1	1	0	1	1	1	1	0
Garden Vegetable Dip (p. 87)	47	3	7	1	87	243	5	39	66	5	11	3	11	3
Pineapple Yogurt Nut Loaf (p. 88)	95	3	16	3	60	144	4	1	1	6	4	3	4	5
Toasty Oat Crackers (p. 86)	19	1	2	1	23	12	1	1	0	2	1	1	0	1

Vegetables

	Calories	Protein gms.	Carbohydrate gms.	Fat gms.	Sodium mgs.	Potassium mgs.	Protein	Vitamin A	Vitamin C	Thiamin	Riboflavin	Niacin	Calcium	Iron
Asparagus Piquant (p. 54)	45	3	10	0	74	367	5	21	67	14	14	9	3	7
Baked Lima Beans with Tomatoes (p. 58)	97	6	15	2	314	315	9	12	24	4	4	4	8	14
Brandied Sweet Potatoes (p. 62)	163	2	33	1	92	310	3	185	61	9	4	3	5	5
Broccoli-Cauliflower Soup (p. 65)	71	6	10	1	337	314	10	20	77	5	15	2	17	3
Cabbage Supreme (p. 59)	73	4	9	3	151	311	6	5	89	5	8	2	13	3
Cheese-Broccoli Bake (p. 58)	65	4	7	3	117	231	6	21	78	4	10	2	10	3
Chilled Asparagus Soup (p. 65)	52	5	9	0	223	348	8	16	47	11	18	6	12	5
Chilled Spinach Bisque (p. 65)	95	5	4	7	514	299	8	121	38	5	10	2	10	9
Chive Creamed Corn (p. 57)	113	4	18	4	203	215	6	9	12	6	7	6	5	4
Company Cabbage (p. 59)	61	1	4	5	203	174	2	25	40	4	2	1	3	2
Creamy Corn and Zucchini (p. 57)	106	6	14	4	107	279	9	10	26	7	11	7	6	3
Crustless Vegetable Quiche (p. 63)	75	6	4	4	97	301	9	82	47	5	12	2	9	11
Curried Potatoes (p. 60)	145	3	21	6	209	494	4	5	44	8	3	9	2	4
Dilled Zucchini (p. 62)	50	2	5	3	38	255	2	11	41	4	6	6	4	3
Fresh Pea Soup (p. 64)	116	8	17	2	306	518	12	48	60	22	15	12	11	14
Herbed Brussels Sprouts (p. 59)	70	4	9	3	118	360	7	12	147	6	8	4	4	8
Herbed Vegetable Combo (p. 52)	39	2	6	2	94	237	2	11	46	5	5	4	3	3
Italian Vegetable Skillet (p. 54)	91	2	10	6	111	220	3	9	54	5	4	2	3	5
Lemon-Glazed Carrots (p. 55)	65	1	9	3	78	320	2	202	18	4	3	3	4	4
Oriental Pea Pods and Spinach (p. 56)	55	3	7	2	247	276	4	64	57	7	7	4	4	10
Parmesan Steamed Vegetables (p. 54)	76	3	8	4	90	337	4	112	96	6	6	3	5	5
Pea and Celery Medley (p. 56)	44	2	7	1	119	192	4	7	22	9	3	4	3	5
Peas and Pods (p. 56)	56	4	9	1	98	210	5	10	28	13	6	8	3	7
Sesame Green Beans (p. 55)	55	2	5	4	183	182	2	10	20	3	4	2	4	3
Spiced Beets and Apple (p. 64)	94	2	18	2	145	396	3	3	44	4	4	3	2	4
Spinach Pie (p. 57)	190	15	7	12	309	336	23	91	26	12	21	3	24	15
Springtime Potatoes (p. 60)	85	3	17	1	153	453	5	3	39	7	6	7	5	4
Stir-Fried Tomatoes and Peppers (p. 52)	44	1	5	2	537	198	2	11	69	3	3	2	2	4
Tangy Green Beans (p. 55)	61	4	7	2	188	172	6	12	18	4	8	2	1	4
Whipped Potato Bake (p. 60)	120	5	14	5	274	351	7	6	26	6	6	6	6	3
Zucchini Oregano (p. 63)	35	1	6	1	57	260	7	12	42	4	5	3	3	3
Zucchini-Stuffed Green Peppers (p. 62)	62	2	9	2	182	378	4	12	181	8	11	12	3	6

RECIPE INDEX

A-B

Apples
  Apple-Banana Frost, 68
  Apple Soufflé, 83
  Bran-Apple Squares, 87
  Fruit with Creamy Banana
    Dressing, 69
  Rainbow Fruit Salad, 68
  Rhubarb-Apple Crush, 90
  Sesame Apple Toss, 69
  Spiced Beets and Apple, 64
  Spiced Fruit Mold, 66
  Waist-Watchers Zabaglione, 86
Asparagus Piquant, 54
Baked Lima Beans with Tomatoes, 58
Bananas
  Apple-Banana Frost, 68
  Banana Logs, 71
  Fizzy Fruit Slush, 90
  Fruit Medley Salad, 71
  Fruit with Creamy Banana
    Dressing, 69
Beef
  Beef and Sprout Sandwiches, 50
  Beef-Broccoli Stir-Fry, 32
  Hungarian Round Steak, 34
  Pared-Down Pizza, 33
  Pepper Beef Stew, 34
  Roast Beef Carbonnade, 32
  Saucy Pepper Burgers, 33
Beets and Apple, Spiced, 64
Berry-Melon Fruit Cup, 84
Beverages
  Cranberry Wine Cooler, 90
  Fizzy Fruit Slush, 90
  Gazpacho Refresher, 88
  Rhubarb-Apple Crush, 90
Bran-Apple Squares, 87
Brandied Sweet Potatoes, 62
Broccoli-Cauliflower Soup, 65
Brussels Sprouts, Herbed, 59
Bulgur Salad, 77
Burgers, Saucy Pepper, 33
Buttermilk-Blue Cheese Dressing, 78

C

Cabbage, Company, 59
Cabbage Supreme, 59
Carrots, Lemon-Glazed, 55
Casseroles
  Chicken Divan, 45
  Pastitsio, 40
  Tuna-Cauliflower Casserole, 41
  Tuna-Zucchini Bake, 42
Cassoulet Soup, 39
Cauliflower Slaw, 78
Cheese
  Banana Logs, 71
  Buttermilk-Blue Cheese Dressing,
    78
  Cheese-Broccoli Bake, 58
  Creamy Cheese Snacks, 87
  Pear and Blue Cheese Salad, 69
Chicken
  Chicken-Asparagus Toss, 75
  Chicken Divan, 45
  Chicken Marengo, 46
  Chicken 'n' Swiss Stacks, 48
  Chicken-Pineapple Salad, 75
  Lemon Broiled Chicken, 47
  Peach Luncheon Salad, 74
  Savory Sauced Chicken, 45
Chilled Asparagus Soup, 65
Chilled Spinach Bisque, 65
Chive Creamed Corn, 57
Chocolate Mousse Meringues, 80
Citrus Salad Toss, 71
Company Cabbage, 59
Confetti Slaw, 78
Cottage Tomato Cups, 74
Crackers, Toasty Oat, 86
Cranberry Orange Mold, 66
Cranberry Wine Cooler, 90
Creamy Cheese Snacks, 87
Creamy Corn and Zucchini, 57
Creamy Strawberry Mold, 66
Crustless Vegetable Quiche, 63
Curried Potatoes, 60

D-I

Desserts
  Apple Soufflé, 83
  Berry-Melon Fruit Cup, 84
  Chocolate Mousse Meringues, 80
  Frozen Orange Mist, 86
  Gingerbread with Lemon Sauce, 83
  Honeydew Ice, 80
  Mandarin Rice Pudding, 85
  Orange Chiffon Dessert, 85

Desserts, continued
  Orange Sponge Cake, 82
  Orange Yogurt Pie, 82
  Peach Torte, 84
  Waist-Watchers Zabaglione, 86
Diet Salad Dressing, 79
Diet Thousand Island Dressing, 79
Dilled Vegetable Medley Salad, 76
Dilled Zucchini, 62
Dip, Garden Vegetable, 87
Eggs
  Crustless Vegetable Quiche, 63
  Spinach Pie, 57
Fish (see also Tuna)
  Fish and Vegetable Bake, 41
  Sole Florentine, 42
Fizzy Fruit Slush, 90
Fresh Pea Soup, 64
Fruit Cup, Berry-Melon, 84
Fruit Medley Salad, 71
Fruit with Creamy Banana
  Dressing, 69
Garden Tuna Salad, 72
Garden Vegetable Dip, 87
Garden Vinaigrette Salad, 76
Gazpacho Refresher, 88
Gingerbread with Lemon Sauce, 83
Green Beans, Sesame 55
Green Beans, Tangy, 55
Ham and Vegetable Roll-Ups, 48
Herbed Brussels Sprouts, 59
Herbed Vegetable Combo, 52
Honeydew Ice, 80
Hungarian Round Steak, 34
Italian Scallop Salad, 72
Italian Vegetable Skillet, 54

J-R

Jambalaya, Shrimp, 44
Lamb
  Cassoulet Soup, 39
  Lamb-Stuffed Squash, 40
  Pastitsio, 40
  Sweet and Sour Lamb, 39
Lemon Broiled Chicken, 47
Lemon-Glazed Carrots, 55
Mandarin Rice Pudding, 85
Marinated Potato Salad, 77
Melons
  Berry-Melon Fruit Cup, 84
  Fruit Medley Salad, 71
  Honeydew Ice, 80
  Rainbow Fruit Salad, 68
Nut Loaf, Pineapple Yogurt, 88

EXERCISE AND IN-FORMATION INDEX